Documenting Sensorimotor Progress

A Pediatric Therapist's Guide

by

Georgia A. DeGangi, Ph.D., OTR, FAOTA

A joint publication of the

Neuro-Developmental Treatment Association (NDTA) and

Therapy Skill Builders, Publishers

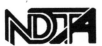

Therapy Skill Builders */*®

a division of
The Psychological Corporation

3830 E. Bellevue / P.O. Box 42050
Tucson, Arizona 85733
1-800-763-2306

Reproducing Pages from This Book

As described below, some of the pages in this book may be reproduced for instructional or administrative use (not for resale). To protect your book, make a photocopy of each reproducible page. Then use that copy as a master for photocopying.

Illustrations were drawn by Carol Knott and are reprinted with the kind permission of Lucy Jane Miller, author of the *Toddler and Infant Motor Evaluation (T.I.M.E™)*, where they also appear.

NUK® is a registered trademark of Gerber Baby Products Col, Fremont, MI 49412.

Velcro® is a registered trademark of Velcro U.S.A., Inc.

The Learning Curve Design is a registered trademark of The Psychological Corporation.

Printed and published in 1994 by

Therapy Skill Builders ✶®
a division of
The Psychological Corporation

3830 E. Bellevue / P.O. Box 42050
Tucson, Arizona 85733
1-800-763-2306

ISBN 0761643117   Catalog No. 4311

10 9 8 7 6 5 4
Printed in the United States of America

For information about our audio and/or video products, write us at: Therapy Skill Builders, a division of The Psychological Corporation, P.O. Box 42050, Tucson, AZ 85733.

Acknowledgments

Many thanks to Martine Ehrenreich, M.S., PT, Mary Goodin, M.Ed., OTR, Esther Horowitz, PT, Marcia Rosenberg, PT, and Nancy Scheiner, M.S., OTR, for treating the cases presented in this manual with their expert therapy skills; to Easter Seals Society of Washington, D.C., and Footsteps Pediatric Physical Therapy in Silver Spring, Maryland, for supporting the case treatments; and to Andrea Santman Wiener, PT, for her assistance in coding the treatment videotapes. Most of all, many thanks are extended to the children and parents who participated in the case profiles presented in this manual. This manual was funded by the NeuroDevelopmental Treatment Association, Inc., and the Cecil and Ida Green Research and Training Institute of the Reginald S. Lourie Center for Infants and Young Children in Rockville, Maryland.

I gratefully acknowledge Lucy Jane Miller's generosity in sharing artwork from her instrument, *Toddler and Infant Motor Evaluation (TIME)* (Miller, L. J., Therapy Skill Builders, Tucson, AZ, 1994), for use in this manual. I would also like to thank Carol Knott, who has blended her remarkable talent in drawing with her skills as an occupational therapist to develop the illustrations for this manual and the *TIME*.

About the Author

Georgia A. DeGangi, Ph.D., OTR, is director of the Cecil and Ida Green Institute for Research and Training at the Reginald S. Lourie Center for Infants and Young Children in Rockville, MD, where she directs research on innovative assessment and treatment strategies. In addition, Dr. DeGangi teaches clinical courses and workshops on the assessment and treatment of infants and young children across the United States, and is on the faculty at Johns Hopkins University.

A recognized leader in the field of neuromotor and sensory integration assessment and treatment in infants and young children, Dr. DeGangi has served on a number of professional boards, including the Neurodevelopmental Treatment Association, the American Occupational Therapy Foundation Research Committee, and the Physical and Occupational Therapy in Pediatrics editorial board. She received her doctorate in applied developmental psychology from the University of Maryland, and an M.S. degree in the education of the moderately to profoundly handicapped from Johns Hopkins University. Dr. DeGangi received her B.S. degree, in occupational therapy, from Boston University.

Contents

Introduction

Increasingly, teachers and therapists are faced with the dilemma of showing that children with special needs benefit from therapeutic and educational intervention. Frequently insurance companies will not authorize payment for therapy services unless a child shows progress from month to month. Parents may wonder how much or how frequently intervention should be provided in order for their child to make progress. Parents may ask whether a particular type of therapy is warranted. Further, referring physicians may question the usefulness of therapy and may be reluctant to refer until there is evidence that treatment is effective.

In response to the growing need to document progress in children with special needs and to demonstrate the effectiveness of therapy programs, *Documenting Sensorimotor Progress: A Pediatric Therapist's Guide* was developed. This text provides a method for documenting changes in infants, preschoolers, and school-aged children with a range of neuromotor problems. It is specifically designed to measure progress after short increments of time, thus allowing the therapist or educator to document changes every few weeks. Since the methods described in this text may be used to chart progress over time, the data obtained from the measures may be used to investigate the benefits of therapy programs.

Documenting Sensorimotor Progress is designed for use by physical therapists, occupational therapists, speech and language communication specialists, special educators, and parents. It has been constructed to help professionals develop specific measures to document progress in movement, functional daily living skills, sensory processing, attention, play, and communication. Since the child with motor problems often has multiple needs—in areas including sensory processing, attention, play, and communication—measures of progress should not be restricted to motor outcomes, even if the therapist is not specifically addressing these other areas in treatment. In fact, some children with more severe motor problems may show gains first in communication, play, attention, or sensory processing, even when therapy is directed toward motor performance. The measures described in this text focus on qualitative components of skills and the processes that impact functional performance.

Documenting Sensorimotor Progress consists of two main sections. Part I describes an overall strategy to use for measuring progress. Part II describes in detail the different areas that may be assessed. Each chapter in Part II includes specific assessment strategies with examples of how measures may be adapted to the needs of different children. Appendix A presents a series of six case examples that may be used as a guide for documenting change. Appendix B discusses methods that may be used for persons interested in conducting their own research.

The assessment strategies described in this manual may be used with children upon referral for intervention as well as for children already receiving intervention. Since the assessment measures presented in Part II are broad in scope, they should be useful for measuring progress with a number of different interventions (e.g., neurodevelopmental treatment, sensory integration, facilitated communication, developmental stimulation). Not only may one evaluate the child's progress over time, but one may use the outlined procedures to evaluate the impact of therapy programs on children. One may assess variables such as frequency, duration, setting, and model of intervention (consultation versus direct hands-on), for example. In this way, the most appropriate therapy and educational program may be devised.

The manual focuses on the needs of motor-impaired children and acknowledges that in most children with delayed motor development, other developmental problems often exist. Usually children with motor problems have abnormal postural tone, delayed reflex maturation, and poor movement quality—with delays in functional skills including fine and gross motor skills, self-care, feeding, and communication. In recent years, it has become evident that children with neuromotor disabilities often have difficulties in learning, paying attention, and with social-emotional skills (Ellenberg and Nelson 1981). Problems associated with motor problems include sensory processing disorders, inattention, perceptual difficulties, immature social-emotional development, and maladaptive play skills.

The methods presented in this book should help professionals streamline their record keeping of everyday observations. Instead of writing a long narrative about what was done in treatment and the child's responses, the therapist or teacher can develop comprehensive checklists, shown in this manual, that may be used readily each time the child is seen for intervention. The checklists encompass easily observable responses to intervention and, therefore, objectify record keeping. As a result, responses may be compared over time for signs of actual change.

The holistic model presented in this manual utilizes a comprehensive assessment that includes neuromotor skills, qualitative movement and posture, tone, self-care and feeding, sensory processing, play behaviors, and other areas affecting functional performance. It goes beyond mere observations of developmental competence. Emphasis is placed on developing sensitive, qualitative observations of daily functional activities. Family concerns are integrated throughout the assessment. By using this holistic, comprehensive assessment model, therapists, parents, and other caregivers may all obtain a more accurate view of how the child functions in the environment.

Documenting Sensorimotor Progress should be useful for parents, particularly in identifying areas of concern for their child. Information in every chapter should help parents understand their child's varying needs. Examples of observations that parents can make about their child in the home, school, or community setting appear throughout this book.

Chapters present background information and details for accurately measuring progress in the following domains:
1. reflex maturation
2. atypical motor and postural control
3. postural tone
4. functional daily living activities
5. emotion regulation, communication, play, and interaction skills
6. sensory processing
7. attention and arousal

Each chapter presents quantifiable methods with which to measure progress in each domain. Six cases, presented in an appendix section, include details on how progress was measured during each short-term therapy program. In each of these six cases, both family and therapists involved in the child's care made observations to document progress.

This manual is intended as a practical guide for therapists, teachers, and parents. The methods described should help these observers document progress more effectively and streamline their record keeping procedures. Because the manual adopts a holistic view of children as they function in the environment, the observations described here should apply to children with a wide range of motor problems.

Part I

PLAN FOR MEASURING CHANGE

Part I describes the steps for measuring change as a result of intervention. The steps include:
- Identifying the most appropriate measures for the child's primary problems; and
- Developing weekly observations to document progress over time.

The procedures described in Part I were piloted on six children to assure their usefulness. These six cases are presented in Appendix A.

1.

DEFINING A MEASUREMENT STRATEGY

The steps described below are designed to assess neuromotor changes over a short period, but they can be modified for children who require intervention longer before change is observed as well.

Step 1: Measure the Child's Primary Problems

Therapists have two basic ways to delineate the child's primary problems for treatment:
- through comprehensive assessment measures
- through the parent interview

Comprehensive child assessment measures are presented in detail in Part II. It is important to involve the parents in the assessment process when attempting to identify the child's primary problems. Typical questions that you might ask a parent include:
- What does your child like to do most of the time? What are the child's favorite types of activities?
- What are some of the things that are hard for your child to do?
- What do you hope that your child will be able to learn to do in the next few months?
- What kinds of things help your child do difficult motor tasks (e.g., positioning, exercises, talking with you, making him interested in a task)?

When families are not available or interested in being interviewed, it may be possible to solicit this information from a teacher or an involved relative or caregiver.

Step 2: Develop Observation Measures to Document Progress Over Time

There are four ways to document change:
- every few months, using test/retest types of measures
- weekly, with observations about specific therapy goals made by the therapist during regular sessions with the child
- semi-weekly, with observations made by the parents regarding the child's progress in areas of greatest concern to them
- intermittently, in a parent (or teacher) interview conducted a designated period of time after the start of the child's therapy

More detail is presented below on how to develop weekly observations for the therapist or parent, and how to measure perception of change. Part II describes many different types of assessments that are useful for both test/retest and weekly observations.

Documenting progress through weekly observations. After completing the initial test for the child, generate a problem list. Since the weekly observations will focus on small changes that the child is making, those things that the therapist, teacher, and parents feel will change in the next few months should be targeted.

Next, develop a weekly observation checklist. It should be completed by the therapist or teacher each time he or she sees the child. Another checklist should be developed for the parents to complete at home once or twice a week if they wish to be involved this way. These observations will serve to document day-to-day (or week-to-week) changes made as a result of therapy. The observations should be very simple, easily observable, and directly related to the problem list and therapy goals identified by the teacher, therapist, and parents.

The observations may involve qualitative movement and posture measures (e.g., "rolls over without severe arching of the back") as well as functional performance measures (e.g., "feeds using a spoon without spilling," "vocalizes during circle time"). When documenting progress, the therapist or teacher simply checks off at the end of the session whether or not the child was able to do a particular skill or function during the session. Those skills not practiced or attempted that day are simply left blank on the checklist. For example, if the therapist does not position the child in standing at all during the treatment session, and one of the observations relates to standing, the therapist leaves blank any observations about how the child did in standing. Reviewing what is or is not checked on the daily log will give you an idea of what was actually done in the intervention. It will also tell you how well the problem list relates to what the child actually needs. The case profiles in Appendix A present numerous examples of daily logs completed by therapists. These logs are easily modified for teachers in classroom settings.

When devising a list of observations to measure, it is a good idea to have more than one represent a given category, if at all possible. The results will tend to be more refined. For example, for the goal,

"Develop graded flexion/extension of the lower extremities in standing," two observations on the log may prove more useful than only one. The first may evaluate lowering the body slowly to squat position to pick up toys on floor; the second may evaluate holding a bear position without assistance while reaching for toys between legs and out to body sides. One can see that these therapist observations are very specific and designed to tap progress in discrete, qualitative motor domains.

The parent observations should be very simple and relate to parent concerns. These may be filled out once or twice a week by the parent(s) during a time that they are observing and playing with their child. If a parent is not available, a teacher or other involved caregiver might make these observations instead. Some skills may be observed incidentally, too, when the parents are carrying, dressing, bathing, or feeding their child.

The wording for the observations must be very clear and easily understood by the parent. Avoid professional jargon. Examples of daily therapy logs completed by the parents are provided in the case profiles in Appendix A. Typical parental observations might include:
"Feeds self with spoon without help."

"Puts down cup with small spill (i.e., no more than one tablespoon lost)." Or, "Puts down cup without a spill."

"Opens door, turning handle or knob."

"Stands alone momentarily."

Because some children with motor problems have many health problems, it is important to document whether the child felt well on the day the observations were made. At the bottom of the checklists, there should be a place to indicate whether the child was healthy that day. Any changes in the therapy program should be noted in a place for comments. For example, a child may be fitted with foot orthotics on an ankle one week, affecting progress.

Measuring the perception of change at the retest. When progress will be measured at the end of a designated period of time, conduct a parent interview to determine the parents' perception of how their child has changed. Questions you might ask include:
* How has your child changed in the past few months?
* What changes have occurred in the following areas?

    —large body movement skills

    —use of hands

    —awareness of body

    —motivation to move

    —posture

    —tone

    —feeding

    —play skills

- Does your child help during dressing, or is your child more comfortable to carry or hold than before?
- Does your child need less help from adults to do things?

Summary

This section presents a general overview of the assessment process. In the next sections, you will find considerable detail on how to measure progress in specific areas that have relevance for the child with motor problems. Refer to Appendix A for examples of specific measures.

Part II

ASSESSMENT STRATEGIES

Part II comprises seven chapters that present detailed assessment strategies for:
- reflex maturation

- atypical motor and postural control

- postural tone and its effect on movement

- functional daily living activities

- emotion regulation, communication, play and interaction skills

- sensory processing

- attention and arousal

Within each chapter, current concepts and theory are reviewed, followed by a description of standardized assessments and qualitative observational measures that should be useful for children with motor handicaps.

2.

REFLEX MATURATION

Many children with neuromuscular dysfunction experience persistence of primitive reflexes and delayed righting and equilibrium reactions. Primitive reflexes may be obligatory or persistent and thus inhibit the development of higher level postural reflexes. More mildly involved children may display remnants of primitive reflexes that interfere with the development of adequate eye-hand coordination, midline integration, and postural control.

Prognostic Significance of Primitive Reflexes

The persistence of primitive reflexes in movement patterns in children with cerebral palsy has been documented as a poor prognostic indicator. The primitive reflexes that have a major impact on motor development include the tonic neck reflexes, positive supporting reaction, Moro, and palmar and plantar grasp reflexes (Molnar and Gordon 1976). These are reviewed below.

Asymmetrical Tonic Neck Reflex. The ATNR is a proprioceptive reflex elicited by movement of the neck musculature and cervical spine. Turning of the head to one side results in extension of the arm and leg on the face side with flexion of the extremities on the skull side (figure 2.1). In the normal infant, the reflex is not obligatory but is often used in initial reaching to the body side. A tonic neck reflex that is obligatory or interferes with function after six months of age represents an impairment of the motor system (Molnar and Taft 1977). Persistence of the ATNR was found to be the most diagnostically useful sign in children with spasticity or dyskinesis (Paine 1964).

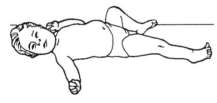
Figure 2.1. The child demonstrates positioning for the asymmetrical tonic neck reflex.

When the ATNR persists and is obligatory, one often sees scoliosis and hip joint subluxation of the skull-side leg. In sitting, the child with an asymmetrical tonic neck reflex will have difficulties staying erect and will often lean severely to one side. A strong ATNR may cause the eyes to fix laterally toward one side. Tracking of the eyes across midline is also very difficult (Bobath 1959). Until the ATNR is integrated, it is difficult for the child to hold the head in midline,

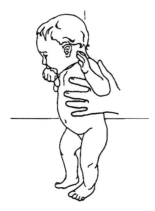

Figure 2.2. The positive supporting reaction is elicited by the ball of the foot touching the floor surface, causing increased extensor tone in the lower extremities.

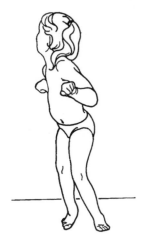

Figure 2.3. In the child with spasticity, toe walking is seen in conjunction with a pattern of extension, adduction, medial rotation, and plantarflexion.

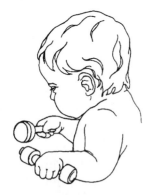

Figure 2.4. The palmar grasp involves a response to a finger or object placed across the baby's palm, resulting in strong flexion or gripping of the fingers.

to grasp and manipulate toys in the midline, roll over, or develop trunk rotation. Remnants of the ATNR will interfere with eye-hand coordination, particularly in maintaining eye contact with midline activities such as catching a ball. Balance is significantly affected when elements of the ATNR remain because of poor trunk rotation and disassociation of the neck and body.

Positive supporting reaction. The positive supporting reaction is described as a mechanism necessary for the maintenance of erect posture (Gilfoyle, Grady, and Moore 1990). The positive supporting reaction is elicited by the ball of foot touching the floor surface, which results in increased extensor tone in the lower extremities (figure 2.2). This reflex normally occurs before four months as a response to weight bearing. Positive supporting may be late in its appearance in children with spastic quadriplegia. If this reflex persists, it results in a stiff, uncontrolled position of the lower extremities, which prevents the establishment of balanced, voluntary standing (Gifoyle, Grady, and Moore 1990). In the child with spasticity, toe walking is seen in conjunction with a pattern of extension, adduction, medial rotation, and plantar flexion (figure 2.3). The child encounters difficulties in transferring the weight forward, and there is a tendency to fall backwards (Bobath 1959).

Moro reflex. The Moro reflex is normal until six months old and occurs in response to such stimulation as tapping the supporting surface while the baby is backlying. The initial response involves abduction and extension of the arms with opening of the fingers, followed by a subsequent movement of the arms into adduction and flexion (Bobath 1959). As the Moro declines, the startle becomes more prominent, a reaction which is predominantly a rapid flexor response (Capute et al. 1978).

Palmar and plantar grasp reflexes. The palmar grasp involves a response to a finger or object placed across the baby's palm, resulting in strong flexion or gripping of the fingers (figure 2.4). The reflex is initially very strong in the newborn and remains present to a minimal degree in six-month-olds. This reflex must fade to allow a functional grasp and release to develop.

The plantar grasp involves flexion of the toes when a finger is placed across the plantar surface just under the toes. Often it does not fade until the infant begins to take weight on the feet at nine to 10 months. A remnant of the plantar grasp may be seen in children who curl their toes when standing.

Automatic and equilibrium reactions. The postural reactions, also known as the automatic and equilibrium reactions, form the base of support upon which voluntary, coordinated, and skilled movements are placed. The normal postural reaction involves automatic adjustments to changes of posture. It involves proximal fixation for the performance of distal movement. The gradual development of the righting reactions underlies the sequence of normal motor development (Scherzer and Tscharnuter 1982).

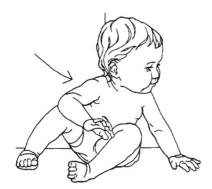

Figure 2.5. The child extends an arm quickly to stop a fall in this demonstration of the lateral protective reaction in sitting.

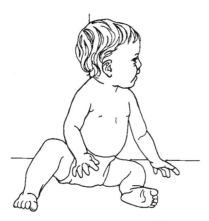

Figure 2.6. As equilibrium reactions are refined, the flexion and extension components are combined to allow rotational movements.

Central control of the neck and trunk develops through maturation of the labyrinthine and optical righting reactions. These reactions return the body posture when there is a loss of the body's orientation, bringing the body into an upright posture. The different righting reactions combine to allow for segmental rolling, sitting up, and crawling.

Protective reactions of the arms and legs develop as a result of weight bearing. They occur when there is a quick displacement or shift in the center of gravity. The arms or legs quickly extend in the direction of the displacement to break the fall (figure 2.5). Their development is dependent upon good trunk stability, and active extension and weight bearing of the extremities.

Equilibrium reactions allow the body to adapt to changes in its own center of gravity to maintain and regain balance. A typical equilibrium reaction in sitting with a lateral displacement includes lateral flexion and rotation of the neck and trunk, with extension and abduction of the extremities away from the displacement. A forward displacement in sitting results in flexion of the lower extremities and extension of the neck and spine, with backward extension of the arms. A backwards displacement in sitting results in forward movement of the neck, shoulders, and arms with leg extension (Bobath 1959).

These equilibrium reactions play an important role in freeing the arms from supporting the body. As equilibrium reactions are refined, the flexion and extension components are combined to allow rotational movements. The trunk can then respond to changes in the center of gravity efficiently, with minimal postural adjustments (figure 2.6). When a child has poor righting and equilibrium reactions, clumsiness, poor balance, and poor gradation of movements are present. Trunk rotation is usually missing in movement transitions. Fine motor skills, particularly bilateral motor control, are often compromised as well.

Assessment of Reflex Maturation

An assessment of reflex maturation should include the following components:

- the presence of primitive reflexes and the degree to which they persist;
- the context in which primitive reflexes occur and their effect on functional movement abilities;
- the development of equilibrium and righting reactions;
- the impact of postural reflexes on fine and gross motor skills.

In addition, one must consider the age at which the primitive reflexes fade, and their evolution over time. In any assessment of reflex maturation, it is important to consider the constellation of postural and movement problems. A single abnormal sign does not constitute a movement disorder, but may reflect a minor irregularity in motor skills.

Suggested assessments for determining reflex maturation include the *Chandler Movement Assessment of Infants* (Chandler et al. 1987), and the *Infant Neurological International Battery (INFANIB)* (Ellison 1994). These assessments should be used in conjunction with an assessment of motor skills (e.g., *Peabody Developmental Motor Scales*). Since abnormal reflex activity or delayed reflex maturation may affect functional movement skills, it is also important to examine qualitative movement skills (see Chapter 5).

The *Chandler Movement Assessment of Infants* (CMAI) is an instrument designed to assess the neuro-motor functions of infants in the first year of life. One intention of the instrument is to monitor the effects of physical therapy on infants and children whose motor skills fall at or below one year of age. The CMAI is a comprehensive assessment of muscle tone, primitive reflexes, automatic reactions, and volitional movements in the first year. Norms are available through the first year of life. Using a percentage agreement described in the manual, individual raters reached 90% agreement. In a study conducted by Harris et al (1984), reliability was fair for the total-risk scores for both interobserver (.72) and test-retest (.76) reliability. Reliability was poor to fair for section-risk scores (i.e., tone, reflexes, and volitional movement subtests) for low- and high-risk infants, with the exception of good reliability for low-risk infants who were administered the volitional movement subtest. (The instrument may be obtained from Lynette Chandler, Movement Assessment of Infants, P.O. Box 4631, Rolling Bay, Washington 98061.)

The *Infant Neurological International Battery (INFANIB)* (Ellison 1994) is an assessment examining the neurological integrity of infants through 18 months of age. It is a 20-item test that includes items from the Milani-Comparetti and Gidoni neurological assessment, French angles (i.e., scarf sign), primitive reflexes, and other observations (e.g., hands open). The test was validated on 365 infants, including 160 normal infants, 134 with transient abnormalities, 21 with hypotonia, and 50 with spasticity. The test contains recommended cut points for classifying infants as abnormal, transiently abnormal or normal in their neurological functions. Reliability coefficients were good for all subscales except the lower extremity items, which were fair.

Summary

In addition to standardized measures, clinical observations of reflex maturation during functional performance are very useful. The presence of obligatory reflexes during daily living tasks (e.g., feeding, dressing) should be observed. Immature postural reflexes may hinder the child's capacity to maintain body positions necessary for self-care and other play and work activities. The next section details some of the ways that these may be observed in various developmental tasks.

3.

ATYPICAL MOTOR AND POSTURAL CONTROL

Atypical movement findings often suggest delayed or abnormal reflex maturation, as well as immature postural reactions and equilibrium responses. These findings may include observations such as asymmetrical tonic neck reflex posturing during reach, hyperextension of the neck with back rounding in sitting, or arching during transitional movements. When qualitative movements or postures are poor, they may suggest a combination of abnormal findings in tone, balance, postural reactions and control, equilibrium responses, and reflex maturation that have important prognostic significance. In this chapter, research findings supporting observations of atypical motor and postural control are described, followed by a description of methods with which to assess qualitative motor observations.

Significance of Atypical Movement Findings

Infants of low birthweight and prematurity comprise one group that has been described with qualitative movement problems. Drillien (1977) introduced the term "transient dystonia" to describe the subtle abnormal neurological findings present in about 50% of infants born prematurely at 2,500 grams or less. This syndrome consists of motor developmental delay, exaggerated manifestation of primitive reflexes, abnormal distribution of muscle tone, and delayed development of postural adjustments. It occurs more frequently in infants with the lowest birth weights. Sixty percent of infants with moderate to severe transient dystonia resolve between eight and 12 months of age with no specific therapeutic intervention. An additional 20% showed equivocal resolution, and the remaining 20% had a definite diagnosis of cerebral palsy.

Transient dystonia may persist well into the second year, especially with babies of early gestational age and very low birth weights. Several investigators (Drillien 1972; Drillien, Thomson, and Burgoyne 1980;

Ellenberg and Nelson 1981) have found a relationship between transient motor dysfunction in infancy, hyperactivity at three years, and learning disabilities at seven years. These reports suggest that the phenomenon of transient dystonia may reflect a more general neurological dysfunction in some children and have important prognostic value.

The specific movement problems observed in children with transient dystonia include neck hyperextension, flexion in the upper extremities, and extensor tonus in the lower extremities. This profile suggests that infants with poor proximal control and abnormal fixation patterns at the pelvic or scapular regions are at risk for later movement and/or learning problems. Based upon this early research, Valvano and DeGangi (1986) explored the prevalence of atypical posture and movement findings in high risk premature infants with suspect neurological signs. The movement problems consisted of arching of the trunk, hyperextension of the neck, rounding of the back in sitting, anterior pelvic tilt, shoulder retraction, fisting of the hands, mirroring of the hands in simple fine motor tasks, and leg stiffness in upright positions. In this study, the performance of the preterm infants was contrasted with full-term babies without motor problems that were from four to 12 months of age. Significantly, the team found that many normally functioning infants display atypical postures and movements when first learning a new motor skill.

Assessment of Atypical Motor Findings

Examination of atypical motor findings in conjunction with observations of motor and neurological functions provides a context of how neuromotor performance impacts function. Typically, qualitative posture and movement findings are not provided for within the standard motor test design. Administration of a motor test that has good reliability and validity is important as a first step.

The *Peabody Developmental Motor Scales* (Folio and Fewell 1983) is a standardized screening instrument for children ranging in age from birth to seven years. It is designed to evaluate both gross and fine motor skills, measuring these behaviors in such a way that emergence and mastery of skills can be documented. Test/retest reliability is .95 for the Gross Motor Scale and .80 for the Fine Motor Scale. Interrater reliability is in the .90s. Content, construct, and concurrent content validity have been established. DLM Teaching Resources (P.O. Box 4000, One DLM Park, Allen, Texas 75002) publishes the test.

The *Toddler and Infant Motor Evaluation (TIME)* (Miller 1994) is designed to measure mild to severe motor problems in children from birth to $3\frac{1}{2}$ years. The test items are developmentally based and include observations of mobility, stability, and motor organization in various positions, including supine, prone, sidelying, sitting, quadruped, kneeling, squat, plantigrade, and standing. The skill levels tested by the *TIME* range from basic floor postures through ambulatory skills. Observations are made of the child in stable postures and as the child moves from one position to another. Responses are elicited to observe equilibrium reactions, trunk rotation, reach and hand use, and other skilled responses (e.g., walking on tiptoes) within the various developmental positions. *TIME* is unique in the way it integrates qualitative posture and movement responses throughout the scoring. For this reason, *TIME* is highly applicable to a wide range of motor problems in infants and toddlers. Each item is illustrated, which allows easy scoring of the child's responses. In addition to providing for the comprehensive evaluation of motor problems in infants and toddlers, *TIME* can also prove useful in measuring progress.

Additionally, a set of clinical observations that may be useful in describing a child's quality of movement and posture were validated on a sample of 193 infants ranging in age from four to 18 months (151 controls and 42 high risk premature infants with mild motor delay) (DeGangi, Berk, and Valvano 1983; Valvano and DeGangi 1986). These observations were noted during administration of the *Bayley Scales of Infant Development, Motor Scale* (Bayley 1969). Observations may be made during administration of other motor scales as well, such as the *Chandler Movement Assessment of Infants* (Chandler et al. 1987) or the *Peabody Developmental Motor Scales* (Folio and Fewell 1983).

Interobserver reliability was attained for the measures presented herein. As reported by Valvano and DeGangi (1986), interclass correlations were .93 for the set of observations for infants ranging in age from birth to 12 months (n = 25).

When evaluating for the presence or absence of the various qualitative movement findings, record data from each set of observations in various developmental positions, including:
- prone
- supine
- sitting
- quadruped and kneeling
- standing

Observe movement quality in the following transitional movements:
- rolling from prone to supine
- rolling from supine to prone
- prone to sitting
- sitting to prone
- supine to sitting
- quadruped to sitting
- sitting to standing

In addition, test fine motor skills and observe upper extremity and hand use items.

The qualitative observations developed by Valvano and DeGangi (1986) for this purpose are presented in table 3.1 and explained below.

Scoring of Qualitative Observations. After observing for the presence or absence of the various qualitative findings listed in table 3.1, total up the number of qualitative observations. Using the data obtained by Valvano and DeGangi (1986), it has been found that seven or more atypical movement problems between the ages of four and 12 months differentiated between infants with motor dysfunction and those without. For infants from 13 to 18 months, six or more atypical movement problems represent a qualitative motor problem.

TABLE 3.1
Qualitative Observations of Posture and Movement

1. *Head posture:*
   a. head rests forward into gravity when vertical (cervical flexion)
   b. chin juts out when vertical (cervical flexion and capital extension)
   c. head rests backward due to low tone when vertical (capital extension and cervical extension)
   d. neck hyperextension with high or changeable tone (capital extension and cervical extension)
   e. neck asymmetries (lateral flexion and rotation)

2. *Trunk posture:*
   a. flexion (spastic)
   b. arching of back
   c. rounding of trunk (in vertical)
   d. asymmetries (lateral flexion and rotation)
   e. mid trunk collapses into gravity

3. *Shoulder girdle:*
   a. scapular elevation
   b. scapular retraction
   c. scapular protraction
   d. scapular asymmetries

4. *Pelvis:*
   a. posterior pelvic tilt
   b. anterior pelvic tilt
   c. pelvic immobility
   d. asymmetries in pelvic tilt

5. *Transitional movements:*
   a. inadequate initiation of movement from head
   b. head does not follow body movement adequately
   c. poor weight shift in trunk
   d. poor weight shift in pelvis
   e. inadequate trunk rotation

TABLE 3.1 (continued)
Qualitative Observations of Posture and Movement

6. *Lower extremity posture:*
   a. exaggerated adduction, inward rotation (not upright)
   b. exaggerated abduction, outward rotation (flaccidity)
   c. extensor thrusting
   d. increased flexion in LE
   e. legs poorly dissociated or show difficulty with reciprocal movement
   f. ataxic movements
   g. stiffness in supporting
   h. withdraws from contact with the floor
   i. poor weight shift onto LE
   j. base too narrow
   k. base too wide
   l. toes in (foot inversion)
   m. toes out (foot eversion)
   n. on toes (plantarflexion)

7. *Upper extremity posture:*
   a. transient fisting with holding posture or movement (not in fine motor tasks)
   b. static fisting with holding posture (not in fine motor tasks)
   c. arms held in abduction in response to movement
   d. posturing of upper extremities during gross movement (flexion at elbows and wrists with fisting of hands typical)
   e. extraneous movement in upper extremities
   f. ATNR pattern
   g. flexion pattern in uppers

8. *Hand use:*
   a. inaccurate reaching with or without tremor
   b. fanning or splaying of fingers during release
   c. mirroring during unilateral task (over one year)
   d. extraneous movement in hands
   e. predominant pronation in grasp
   f. transient fisting of uninvolved hand in unilateral task
   g. static fisting of uninvolved hand in unilateral task

Summary

By using a variety of clinical observations of posture and movement in combination with assessments of tone, reflex maturation, and functional movement capacity, the therapist will find it possible to gather relevant data regarding the neuro-motor status of a child. These observations may then be used in developing appropriate treatment goals and measures to document progress.

4.

POSTURAL TONE AND ITS EFFECT ON MOVEMENT

The concept of muscle tone is an important one because it is used as a basis for diagnosis of neurological impairment, and is often a justification for the need to intervene therapeutically. Muscle tone is always affected in infants and children with neurological abnormality. Infants with tonal abnormalities have been found to be more likely to develop later motor handicaps (Ellenberg and Nelson 1981). It has been cautioned, however, that tonal abnormalities observed in the first year of life may be variable and difficult to quantify in terms of pathology until after one year of age (Amiel-Tison and Grenier 1983).

Since observations of tone during and after therapy are often used as an indicator of the child's responsiveness to intervention, an understanding of the concept of tone and how it may be objectively measured is important. In the following sections, muscle tone and postural tone are defined. The impact of tone on movement is described and the various types of tonal disturbances are presented. A model for conceptualizing tone is provided. It is followed by a discussion of methods to assess tone objectively.

Definition of Muscle Tone

Tone has been defined in many different ways. Bobath has described tone as an "ongoing physiological adaptation . . . a condition of readiness. Tone is not merely a condition of the muscles, but of the entire neuromuscular apparatus." (Bobath 1985). Others have referred to tone as resistance to passive and active movement of the limbs and body (Amiel-Tison and Grenier 1983; Brazelton 1984). Andre-Thomas and associates (1960) defined passive tone as involving extensibility, the capacity of the muscle to be lengthened, and the lack of resistance to passive movement. Passive muscle tone was considered inversely proportional to extensibility. Tone has also been conceptualized in terms of the properties of muscles (e.g., the amount of stiffness or laxity in response to resistance to stretch).

The concept of tone is very complex. Muscle tone may be thought of in terms of biomechanics and neuromuscular mechanisms (Gordon 1990). The biomechanical aspects of tone affect joint posture and the resistance of muscles to stretch. The neuromuscular aspects of tone relate to the intrinsic stiffness of muscles and neural control over reflexive and voluntary muscle activity. More recently, attention has shifted toward the impact of motor plans and programs on tone, and differences in unskilled versus skilled automatic movement (Schmidt 1991; Brooks 1986).

Muscle tone may be considered dynamic and an important component of normal posture and movement. Normal muscle tone is high enough to support the body against gravity, yet low enough to allow movement. The distribution of tone changes over the course of development. Neonates tend to exhibit lower tone in the trunk and increased tone in the extremities. However, with motor maturity, muscle tone becomes higher proximally, providing a stable base upon which skilled distal movements are founded (DeGangi, Berk, and Valvano 1983). In addition, tone is changeable in response to sensory stimulation, task demands, the intention of the mover, and the level of motor maturity over development (Scherzer and Tscharnuter 1982).

Definition of Postural Tone

The concept of muscle tone has expanded to include "postural tone." Postural tone involves redistribution of muscle tone within the entire body in response to changes in body position, alignment, or shifts in the center of gravity. Postural tone development allows for refinements in postural stability, development of muscle co-contraction, and the grading of coordinated movements. Postural tone develops as a result of:

- normal postural alignment and muscle tone
- tactile-proprioceptive and vestibular feedback mechanisms
- reflex maturation, allowing for postural adjustments and balance
- central nervous system maturation (e.g., axonal myelinization)
- the development of motor plans and motor programs

Impact of Tone on Movement

In order to have normal movement, one must have normal postural alignment and muscle tone. Muscle tone should feel steady and be of moderate intensity if performance is to be smooth and precise (Bobath 1959). Tone provides an ongoing readiness of the periphery to move and is, therefore, related to coordinated activity (Bobath 1971). Invisible shifts of muscle tone throughout the body provide for postural adaptations. Muscle tone changes precede movement and are automatic and dynamic. The Bobaths have described normal muscle tone as co-existing with a normal postural reflex mechanism (Bobath and Bobath 1964).

Tonal disturbances. Muscle tone disturbances and impaired coordination are common among children with cerebral palsy (Bobath 1971; Bobath and Bobath 1984). Marked differences in muscle tone are associated with stereotypic movement patterns and postures in children with cerebral palsy. The Bobaths have described abnormal tone as a "release" phenomenon related to the release of abnormal reflex activity from cortical inhibitory control (Bobath and Bobath 1952, 1956; Bobath 1971). The concept of "release" from the central nervous system (CNS) is oversimplified. It does not consider the capacity to motor plan, program, and execute movement (Brooks 1986; Marsden 1982).

Hypotonicity is defined as a lack of resistance in the muscle, or as a floppiness associated with the child's movements. Postural instability and incoordination, as well as hypermobility of the joints, are common problems of the hypotonic child. Many children with learning disabilities exhibit mildly decreased muscle tone.

Hypertonicity occurs when there is too much tension or resistance to passive movement. Excessive stiffness or muscle co-contraction are present. Spasticity is often considered part of the hypertonicity and involves a constellation of clinical symptoms such as clonus, and increased flexor reflexes. Muscle weakness often underlies hypertonicity.

Illingworth (1966) has described some of the movement patterns associated with muscle tone disturbances seen in infants with cerebral palsy. Increased abduction in the hips is representative of hypotonia, while decreased abduction of the hips is observed with hypertonicity. Decreased ankle dorsiflexion is very common in spasticity. Excessive extensor tone may be evident when held in ventral suspension. In pull to sit, the child may move to stand rather than sit if there is trunk and hip extensor spasticity.

Often infants who later develop definite neurologic signs, including abnormal reflex activity and hypertonicity, go through an early stage of hypotonicity (Molnar and Taft 1977; Bly 1983). The transition from hypotonicity to hypertonicity frequently occurs at around six months in infants with neurologic damage (Paine 1969). Initially hypertonicity is generally seen in the lower extremities. A marked discrepancy in muscle tension between the upper and lower extremities should be investigated. In addition, hypertonicity in both upper and lower extremities in the newborn is not as unfavorable a prognostic sign as the observation of hypotonicity (Rosenblith and Anderson 1968). When hypotonicity is present, decreased tone in the trunk is considered more serious than hypotonia of the extremities (Dargassies 1972).

A Model for Conceptualizing the Interaction of Tone and Movement

One way to conceptualize the dynamic nature of postural tone is to consider it in relation to phases of movement and posture. **Movement** involves the starting and stopping of the body and its parts in space. **Posture** is the maintenance of a stable body position to allow for either weight bearing or holding the trunk or limbs in space. Essentially there are three phases of movement and posture:

1. Initiation of movement to assume a body posture or to move the extremity in space

2. Sustainment of body or extremity posture

3. Movement out of one posture in order to assume another, or to allow for a functional skill

This last phase involves many of the same processes that occur during initiation of movement. Some of the components of movement as they relate to these three phases are outlined below.

Initiation of Movement

Consider:

Speed, power, and force of movement. Is speed slow in the first phases of movement due to too much muscle co-contraction, postural fixation, or underlying muscle weakness? Is speed different once child has first initiated movement (i.e., quick and explosive)? Is the movement quick, accompanied by a great deal of force, or is there little power? Is the movement sluggish or explosive in nature?

Quality of movement. Is movement fluid? What components of normal movement are present (flexion, extension, rotation)? Does child rely on more primary patterns of movement (i.e., flexion or extension)?

Weight shift through movement. Are there gradations of weight shifts through the movement? Is the weight shift sustained? Is there postural holding over body parts during the weight shift, or is there collapse over the supporting extremity and trunk?

Weight-bearing phase in attaining final postures. Is there postural stability, or do postural fixations interfere with adequate stability? What is the base of support? Where is the center of gravity?

Motor planning components. Is there reliance on visual, verbal, or physical cues to initiate movement? What motivates the movement (e.g., task)? Are obstacles and furniture surfaces negotiated? Is the transition efficient, or does it involve more movements than necessary?

Sensory components. Is there toleration of contact on different body surfaces on the floor or furniture? Are there hyper- or hyposensitivities to movement (i.e., fear of moving into a position, or sensitivities to

INNOVATIVE THERAPY NETWORK
11270 Washington Blvd.
Culver City, CA 90230

rotation of the neck in space)? Does the child have a strong preference for certain types of movement or postures (e.g., bouncing; upright)? Is there awareness of body limbs and their position (i.e., are extremities caught under the body without awareness)?

Consistency. Are there differences in the way in which movement is initiated in different positions, depending upon the context and task, etc.?

Sustainment of Posture

Consider:

Quality of posture once attained. **Alignment:** What is alignment of trunk, pelvis, and shoulder girdle? Are extremities placed properly for weight bearing or other functions? **Dynamic weight shifts:** Are there weight shifts, once position is attained? Are there postural fixations to hold the position? **Weight-bearing surface:** What is the base of support? Are the weight bearing surfaces effectively placed? What is the body position in relation to the supporting surface?

Duration of holding posture. Is posture stable enough to be maintained while engaged in task? Is position held too long (i.e., may there be low motivation to move)?

Frequency of posture in movement repertoire. Is the posture a familiar one that is used consistently, or is it emergent?

Position for function. Does the position lend itself to function? What functions are limited by the choice of position?

Movement Out of Posture

Consider:

Transition out of posture. Leaving a supporting surface to move into another position or to engage in functional skill. Consider speed, power, and force of movement.

Purposefulness of movement. Was the movement intended, or was there involuntary reflex or movement activity? Was the child motivated to move?

Movement into posture to allow for function. What factors interfere with engagement in skilled functions (i.e., feeding, hand use, gait)?

Assessment Techniques to Quantify Tone

Tone may be measured through observations of positional restrictions or by palpations of tone while the individual is moved passively by the examiner. For example, extensibility of a muscle may be evaluated through range of motion as a muscle group is lengthened, and by palpating the amount of resistance encountered while performing a given movement. Passive muscle tone may also be assessed by shaking a limb to elicit quick alternate muscle stretches while at the same time observing the range and movement of the distal portion of the limb in relation to the point of support. Active tone may be assessed by the amount of recoil observed in a muscle after a limb has been passively lengthened by the examiner. Active tone may also be observed through static postures assumed by the individual, strength of reflexes, and coordinated movements. Therefore, active tone may be measured by observing the individual's spontaneous movement and posture choices, the number of positions assumed in a period of time, and the speed of movement transitions.

Objectivity in assessing tone has been an ongoing problem for therapists and doctors. In a recent study, for example, low reliability was obtained in overall ratings of tone in a clinical setting where six physical therapists rated muscle tone using individual assessment methods (Kathrein 1990). Consistent terminology and methods of assessing tone are needed. The methods for assessing tone suggested in this section should be used in conjunction with standardized tests (e.g., *Chandler Movement Assessment of Infants* and the *Infant Neurological International Battery*).

Observations of day-to-day changes in tone. In examining the effects of NDT handling techniques, it is important to document how the child's tone changes as a result of handling within a session and over time. The child may be observed before and after each treatment session to examine changes that occurred on a given day. What is more meaningful, however, is noting how well the child consolidates the changes in tone over time. A child may be observed by the parent in everyday activities to determine changes in areas related to tone. The therapist should also observe similar types of responses during sessions. This will provide validity—that is, the parent and therapist both agree that the child has shown positive change in tone. Observations may include:

- improved mobility (e.g., when placed on the floor in a particular position, such as supine or sitting, the child moves out of it to a desired position)
- better holding of the body against gravity (e.g., when standing up at the table, the child does not lean into the furniture; or when sitting at the table engaged in fine motor tasks, the child does not lean on the forearms)
- improved postural alignment (e.g., when sitting on a therapy bench, the child keeps the feet well grounded on the floor but does not depend on his hands for support)
- less stiffness of the limbs (e.g., when dressed or bathed by the parent, the child is easier to work with, so that it takes less time to do these daily tasks)

There are many examples of how tone may be observed functionally through meaningful movement activities. The case profiles in Appendix A present more examples of how these activities were typically observed both by parents and therapist.

Reliability of observations. In order to assure objectivity in scoring observations, the child's responses should be videotaped and rated by two observers to determine interobserver agreement. If videotaping is not possible, another therapist may independently score the child's responses.

Procedures. **Select two movement patterns or transitional movements that the parent and therapist agree need work and reflect the child's tone problem.** For example, it may be head lifting in prone, sitting up from supine, standing up from sitting on bench, focusing eyes on target in midline, walking from one point to another, or reaching for a toy. Describe the two movement patterns precisely, with specific criteria, in order to qualify an improved response. For example, if the child has high tone with an inability to shift weight over the pelvis, better tone may be observed when the child can sit on a therapy bench and lift a foot to have his sock put on.

Define exactly how you will position the child each time you measure the movement. For example, the child may be sitting in an adapted chair while you measure head lifting. Define the final end position and how you will measure it. For example, when the child lifts his head, the eyes are looking straight ahead at a target on the wall, the neck is aligned in neutral without evidence of neck hyperextension.

Develop a procedure for motivating the child's movements for each position. For example, select a favorite toy that holds the child's interest. For some children, the stimulus used to motivate the movement may change over the course of the project. Generally, the toy or activity should be novel and not be used for any other purpose during the course of treatment (i.e., during treatment or home program) except for eliciting baseline and post-test measures. Describe the stimuli that will be used to elicit each of the movements.

Observe frequency and duration of movements during spontaneous free play. How often and how long a child holds certain positions—or moves in and out of position—gives information about how the child uses his tone. Allow the child to explore on his own for three minutes before and after the session. Place two interesting toys on the mat, using the same two toys at the beginning and end of the session. Check the number of times that each movement is performed, or how long certain positions are held.

Summary

Postural tone may be conceptualized in many different ways. This section presents a model designed for everyday observations of tone. Since such observations are individualized for each particular child, the reader is referred to the case profiles in Appendix A for concrete information about how tone may be measured in easily observable behaviors. The children participating in the pilot study represent different types of motor handicaps and tone disturbances, so the examples are fairly representative of cases seen in typical practice.

5.

FUNCTIONAL DAILY LIVING ACTIVITIES

Gaining functional independence in daily living skills is a major goal of neurodevelopmental treatment. Self-care or activities of daily living encompass a wide range of tasks, including feeding, dressing, hygiene, sleeping, toileting, play, work, and mobility in the environment. These tasks give life regularity and meaning. Acquiring these skills is a necessary component toward independent living, a healthy adaptation to the environment, and emotional self-reliance. The way in which a person engages in these various tasks is greatly affected by cultural norms and standards.

The performance of functional activities is intrinsically related to the child's drive to engage in purposeful activity and the capacity to adapt to environmental demands. In order for individuals to become independent in functional daily living activities, they must be able to do the following:

- sequence the components of the activity, a skill that requires both motor and cognitive planning

- integrate the motor, perceptual, sensory, cognitive, and communication aspects of the task components into a daily living routine

- engage in purposeful or intentional activity

- assert autonomy and competence

- interact and communicate with caregivers, family, and others while engaged in purposeful activity

- interact and adapt to environmental and task demands

- derive satisfaction from the intrinsic reinforcement related to a given daily living activity

- generalize select skills from one domain to another and integrate these skills into a meaningful activity

What is the process that helps a child gain functional independence in daily living skills? Simple repetition of attained skills only helps the child do a particular skill within a given context. What the child needs, however, is to learn to adapt to increasing or changing environmental and task demands. Only then can the child integrate developmental sequences into purposeful, goal-directed sequences that occur. For example, a child may learn a simple developmental action, such as scooping with a spoon. This feeding action becomes purposeful when the child must adapt to different feeding situations and different foods. Some elements to consider adding to the activity in this example to make it more purposeful to the child might be:

- understanding the rules of eating in a social situation (e.g., don't throw food)
- socializing with family members while eating
- appreciating routines and sequences that happen at mealtime (e.g., setting table, clean-up time)
- managing different food, tableware, and seating requirements (e.g., scooping different textures and consistencies of food with different-sized spoons; sitting in different types of chairs while eating)

A skill becomes consolidated when the child can modify the actions in accordance with situational, task, environmental, and social demands. Coordinated movements required for one action or skill must be modified to suit diverse circumstances.

A Theoretical Framework for Functional Performance

"Occupational performance" is a recent theoretical construct with considerable application and meaning toward the development of functional daily living skills (Kielhofner 1985). Motor actions may be divided into two fundamental categories:

- the movement of the body and objects
- the sequencing of organized actions

This framework considers the influence and interaction of human and nonhuman environmental factors on a child's competence.

Occupations are considered environmental transactions, and they include self-care, work, and play. These skills form the basis for exploration and mastery of the environment (Gilfoyle, Grady, and Moore 1990). These skills give life experiences meaning and motivate the person to engage in goal-directed, purposeful occupations. Within this model of occupational performance, the values, interests, habits, routines, and skills of the child are considered as they occur in the environment.

One may look at the occupations that are meaningful for infants and children by observing certain performance skills. These include:

- motor control—mobility, exploration of environment, and non-verbal communication

- sensory modulation—awareness of changes in environment, attention and arousal
- adaptive coping—taking care of oneself in new environments
- sensorimotor development—concepts, memory, and problem solving
- daily living skills—eating, dressing, etc.
- play as a purposeful activity

These skills facilitate functional performance in young children (Gorga 1989).

Sequence of Developing Functional Performance Skills

Daily living skills are acquired in a generally predictable order. This sequence, derived from Reilly's (1974) play sequences, is described below.

First stage. In the first stage, the child exhibits intentionality, curiosity, and a motivation to explore. First the child explores objects and new experiences. People evoke curiosity, and novel events arouse interest. During this stage, we see the child exploring the characteristics of objects involved in daily care. For example, the child may play with food, articles of clothing, or bath water to experiment with the qualities of these mediums while testing out what can done with them using simple motor actions.

Second stage. This phase focuses on competence. Actions are repeated and newly acquired skills are practiced. Modifications of routines are attempted. This experimentation helps the child develop more efficient ways of doing skills. The child attends to the important features of the skill that help in its acquisition. Depending upon the skill, the child may attend to movement components, qualities of objects, social rules and behaviors of other people, or characteristics of the environment.

Third stage. The last phase of skill acquisition involves mastery. Skills are repeated and practiced with increasing environmental demands. Mastery involves both intrinsic and extrinsic motivation. The child becomes aware of his own abilities and begins to self-evaluate his effectiveness in completing certain tasks. It is during this phase that the child learns to self-correct actions, relying less on others for help. During the mastery stage, the child experiments with the environment to see what happens when it is changed. The child may play dress-up games, or imitate his parent cooking or housekeeping.

Assessment of Functional Performance

The *Vineland Adaptive Behavior Scales* (Sparrow, Balla, and Cicchetti 1984) may be used to assess the various sub-domains within the area of functional performance. The test is a revision of the *Vineland Social Maturity Scale* by Edgar A. Doll. The scales are available in three versions: Interview Edition, Survey Form; Interview Edition, Expanded Form; and Classroom Edition. The test was designed to assess personal and social sufficiency of individuals with and without handicaps from birth to adulthood. It is easily administered through an interview by a caregiver or other person who knows the client well. It measures adaptive behavior in four domains: communication (receptive, expressive, written), daily living skills (personal, domestic, community), socialization (interpersonal relationships, play and leisure time, coping skills) and motor skills (gross and fine motor). This measure is a reliable, valid diagnostic tool. American Guidance Service, Inc. (Circle Pines, Minnesota 55014) publishes this test.

Feeding and oral-motor functions may be assessed using the *Oral-Motor/Feeding Rating Scale* (Jelm 1990). This scale is designed for children from one year through adulthood. It includes sections on oral-motor and feeding patterns, areas related to feeding (i.e., adaptive equipment, sensitivity), respiration/phonation and gross and fine motor function. The test is designed as a rating scale to document qualitative difficulties in oral-motor and feeding skills. Therapy Skill Builders publishes this test. (P.O. Box 42050, Tucson, Arizona 85733).

Daily Therapy Observations to Document Change in Functional Skills

During the therapy program, daily observations may be made by the therapist and/or parent to document changes throughout the course of treatment. Because self-care activities occur every day in the course of everyday tasks, they are observed easily by parents. Some suggestions for structuring observations are presented in this section. In some cases, both therapist and parent observations are presented. Table 5.1 presents examples of observations that may be used in measuring feeding skills. Table 5.2 presents observations of mobility skills and table 5.3 depicts examples for dressing.

Summary

These types of everyday observations may be designed for any behaviors that cause concern for the family and child. Once goals have been targeted, each skill should be broken into component parts. It should be noted that some children do best when they complete the last step of the sequence (i.e., pull zipper up after aligned in placket). Some tasks, however, lend themselves better to the child performing the first step (i.e., tying first knot in shoe tying) because of the complexity of the steps involved. The reader is referred to the clinical cases presented in Appendix A for other examples.

TABLE 5.1
Feeding Observations

Observations Conducted by the Therapist:

1. Normalization of hypersensitivities to touch around lips and in mouth
   a. Tolerates touch around lips: Y   N
   b. Tolerates touch in mouth (without gagging, crying, vomiting):   Y   N

2. Inhibition of gag reflex
   a. Nipple of bottle can be placed in mouth without gag: Y   N
   b. Spoon can be placed firmly on tongue without gag: Y   N

3. Improve lip closure
   a. Closes lips around nipple, maintaining a good seal: Y   N

4. Improve suck and swallow
   a. Sucks continuously on bottle during feeding: Y   N
      Duration of time that sucks continuously _____
   b. Amount of fluid ingested:
      Duration of feed _____
      Amount ingested _____
   c. Evidence of vomiting during session: Y   N
      Frequency _____

5. Inhibition of neck and trunk hyperextension during feeding
   a. Neck hyperextension observed when held in supported sitting: Y   N

6. Improve hand-to-mouth behaviors
   a. Hands hold bottle: Y   N
   b. Brings hands to mouth: Y   N

Observations Conducted by Parents:

Case #1:

1. Tolerates touch around lips: Y   N

2. Tolerates touch in mouth (without gagging, crying, vomiting):   Y   N

3. Nipple of bottle can be placed in mouth without gag: Y   N

4. Spoon can be placed firmly on tongue without gag: Y   N

5. Closes lips around nipple without losing milk: Y   N

6. Length of time to drink bottle: _____

   Amount ingested _____

7. Vomiting during feeding: Y   N

   Frequency _____

   After feeding?   Y   N

8. Hands hold bottle: Y   N

9. Brings hands to mouth: Y   N

continued

TABLE 5.1 (continued)
Feeding Observations

Case #2:

1. Feeds self with spoon without help:	Y	N
—with minimal help:	Y	N

2. Stirs spoon in cup:	Y	N

3. Puts cup down with small spill (i.e., no more than 1 tablespoon lost):	Y	N
Puts cup down with no spill:	Y	N

TABLE 5.2
Observations of Mobility Skills

Case #1:

1. Improve mobility on floor:
   a. Rolls from back to stomach toward left side: Y N
   b. When left by herself on mat for three minutes, will roll over
      if encouraged: Y N
      How many times? _____

Case #2:

1. Improve trunk rotation in various developmental positions:		
a. Gets in and out of child-sized chair using trunk rotation:	Y	N

2. Improve ambulation skills:		
a. Stands at furniture without leaning into it:	Y	N
b. Pushes cart while walking without leaning trunk on handles:	Y	N

TABLE 5.3
Dressing Observations

1. Ties shoes		
—Ties first knot:	Y	N
—Forms bunny ear loops:	Y	N
—Crosses bunny ear loops:	Y	N
—Ties bunny ear loops in knot:	Y	N

2. Buttons buttons		
—On clothing on self:	Y	N
—On doll or other person:	Y	N
Size: Small ($1/2$") _____ Medium ($3/4$") _____		

3. Zips zipper on jacket		
—Aligns zipper into placket:	Y	N
—Pulls zipper up all the way to top using left hand:	Y	N
—Needs reminder to hold with right hand:	Y	N

6.

EMOTION REGULATION, COMMUNICATION, PLAY, AND INTERACTION SKILLS

Many children with neuromotor dysfunction experience difficulties in affective expression, gestural and verbal communication, play and interaction skills. This section presents an overview of the domain of emotion regulation, communication, and play and interaction skills. Various clinical observations and assessments are reviewed that may be used in detecting difficulties in these areas.

Emotion Regulation

Emotions exert a powerful impact on our experience of the world. They motivate us to act and affect the way in which we interact with others and our environment. Emotions provide life experiences with meaning. By guiding our thoughts and actions, emotions have a regulatory function, thus helping us acquire adaptive behavior patterns (Izard 1971).

Emotional expression provides a window into an individual's internal experience of the world. By observing the emotions expressed by others, we can learn how people perceive themselves and others, what interests them, and how well they are able to self-regulate when presented with challenging situations. Emotions mediate the individual's capacity to adapt or respond to a variety of experiences. The child with neuromuscular dysfunction may experience difficulty regulating emotions.

Perceptual problems in recognizing facial expressions or in discriminating gestural or vocal expressions are common in children with neuromuscular dysfunction. They may not be able to discern the signals and cues that other people are sending them. Some children experience difficulties understanding limits because they have not recognized the causal relationship between their actions and the outcomes they produce, or they may not evaluate situations effectively. Low motivation may affect the child's drive to move or to learn new skills. Motivation is related to the child's state of attention, emotion regulation, and capacity to plan and monitor his own actions. Because postural and facial muscles are affected by abnormal tone, the child with neuromotor difficulties may not be able to communicate emotions effectively by gesture or facial expression.

Communication, Play, and Interactions

In the following section, a model is presented for understanding communication, play, and interactions. It is based upon the developmental-structuralist model described by Greenspan (1979, 1989) and Greenspan and Lourie (1981).

Homeostasis: Engagement and attachment. The infant's first task is to take interest in the world and regulate himself. It is generally recognized that self-regulatory mechanisms are complex and develop as a result of physiological maturation, caregiver responsivity, and the infant's adaptation to environmental demands. In the early stages of development, the caregiver soothes the young infant when distressed and facilitates sleep/wake cycles and states of alertness (Kopp 1987).

As the child develops, the caregiver attaches affective meanings to situations, and provides social expectations and values related to specific emotional responses (Kopp 1989). The capacity for engagement and attachment has to do with both physical capacities of the infant, such as the ability to modulate and process sensory experiences (including visual, auditory, tactile, olfactory, vestibular, proprioceptive), and the ability to coordinate simple motor actions, such as reaching for the caregiver's face. The development of action schemes (e.g., vocalizations, self-distractions, or other motor responses), cognitive organization (e.g., representational thinking, self-monitoring) and motivation, and external support from caregivers have been proposed as key elements in attainment of emotion regulation. This in turn is a key element in the development of self-regulation (Weissbluth 1989).

Intentionality and communication. This stage of homeostasis and attachment is followed by the development of intentional organized behaviors. Some of the important milestones of this stage include the development of reciprocal interactions, purposeful communication, an understanding of causal relationships, and development of self-initiated organized behaviors. There is an increase in interactive signalling through gestures. A hallmark of this stage of development is that the infant learns to modify his own actions in response to events in the environment. By interacting with others, the infant discovers that specific actions obtain certain results. The infant also learns that he can control other people's actions. During this stage, the caregiver plays an important role in helping the infant attach meanings to his actions and the environment. Babies begin to learn intentionality through everyday routines and through events that have special meaning, such as going outside or sitting in the high chair (Lewis 1987).

Representational meanings. The last major stage of emotional development involves representational capacity. The toddler shifts from organizing behavioral patterns to abstracting the functional meaning of human and inanimate objects. At this level, the child develops the ability to label feelings and emotions and elaborate upon them. Representational play is motivated by inner desires, issues, and anxieties (Bettelheim 1987). Children dramatize feelings related to dependency, pleasure, assertiveness, curiosity, anger, empathy, and other important themes. This stage, occurring between 18 and 30 months of age, is an important one whereby the child can create mental images that can be manipulated. This is evidenced through his pretend play and his functional use of language. The child is able to attribute affective meanings to objects, people, and events. He can also ascribe affective meanings to his own feelings.

Play of Children with Neuromotor Handicaps

Recent research suggests that children with handicaps demonstrate different play behaviors when compared to their peers without handicaps. Children with motor handicaps are restricted in their play because of difficulties in exploring the environment, combining objects, and interacting with adults and peers. These children may be dependent on others to help them play, thus making them more passive in nature (Greenberg and Field 1982; Jennings et al. 1985). When the child is also mentally retarded, play is restricted in representational themes with reduced language and more constricted use of toy materials (Li 1981).

Assessment Strategies

The parents' concerns at the outset of therapy should be assessed through the use of the checklist in this section that contains questions related to sleep, self-calming, feeding, communication and language, and emotional responses. The checklist is structured in such a way that it is possible to determine the extent of the problem and changes in behavioral patterns over development. Table 6.1 (see page 40) presents the clinical observations for the domains of homeostasis and play and interaction behaviors for use with infants and young children. Table 6.2 (see page 41) presents observations for auditory processing and communication.

Three or more affirmative responses in any one category, such as the "play and interactions" area, may indicate a problem.

TABLE 6.1
Clinical Observations of Homeostasis and Play and Interactions

Homeostasis:

1. Difficulty calming self when upset or stressed.

2. Frequently irritable and fussy.

3. Unable to wait for food or toy without falling apart.

4. Can't change from one activity to another without distress.

5. Demands company constantly.

6. Is not sleeping through night and has difficulty falling asleep.

7. Requires extensive help to fall asleep.

Play and interactions:

1. Avoids eye contact, turns away from human face, prefers objects and toys (over 9 months).

2. Does not appear happy and content.

3. Does not initiate interactions with caregiver; parent must woo infant/child constantly.

4. Does not interact reciprocally (back-and-forth exchanges with caregiver).

5. Does not play with toy telephone or symbolic play games such as feeding a doll by 18 months.

6. Breaks toys and other things destructively.

7. Has difficulty separating from parents, school, or babysitter.

8. Will go to anyone, including strangers (over 2 years).

9. Does not respond to limit setting or discipline.

10. Is self-abusive.

11. Must have total control of environment—"runs the show."

12. Has difficulty getting over temper tantrums.

TABLE 6.2
Clinical Observations of Auditory Processing and Communication Problems

Auditory processing:

1. Does not follow simple instructions.

2. Is not interested in pointing to pictures or objects.

3. Seems overly sensitive to sound; startles or is distressed by loud sounds (i.e., vacuum, door bell, or barking dog).

4. Is confused about the direction of sounds.

5. Likes to make loud noises.

Communication:

1. No, or very little, vocalizing or babbling (six to 12 months).

2. Has a limited variety of consonant sounds, particularly for sounds /p/, /b/, /m/, /n/, /d/, /t/, /w/.

3. Uses fewer than five to seven true words consistently by 18 months.

4. Repeats or echoes previously heard words, phrases, or sentences (over 18 months).

5. Uses extreme repetition of familiar words or phrases (over two years).

6. Is not combining two words to convey meanings by two years, or three- to four-word sentences by three years.

Assessment Measures

A number of assessment procedures are available to measure emotion regulation, communication, play and interaction skills. These are described in this section.

Emotion regulation. One standardized assessment that is useful in quantifying both child and parent characteristics is the *Parenting Stress Index* (Abidin 1986). It is well-standardized and measures both child characteristics and dimensions of parent stress. The 47 items within the Child Domain measure adaptability, how accepting the child is, how demanding, mood, distractibility/hyperactivity, and how satisfying the child is to parent. The 54 items in the Parent Domain measure depression, attachment, restrictions of role, sense of competence, social isolation, relationship with spouse, and parent health. The instrument is self-administered by the parent and can be completed within 10 to 15 minutes. For parents who are unable to read, the scale may be completed with an examiner. The PSI Manual reported reliabilities ranging from .62 to .70 for the Child Domain and from .55 to .80 for the Parent Domain. The reliability for the Total Stress Score is .95. Test-retest reliability over three-week and three-month intervals were also quite high. The PSI is available through Pediatric Psychology Press (320 Terrell Road West, Charlottesville, VA 22901).

The *Vineland Adaptive Behavior Scales* (Sparrow, Balla, and Cicchetti 1984) is a revision of the Vineland Social Maturity Scale by Edgar A. Doll. The scales are available in three versions: Interview Edition, Survey Form; Interview Edition, Expanded Form; and Classroom Edition. The test was designed to assess personal and social sufficiency of individuals, with and without handicaps, from birth to adulthood. It is easily administered by interview by a caregiver or other person who knows the client well, measuring adaptive behavior in four domains: communication (receptive, expressive, written), daily living skills (personal, domestic, community), socialization (interpersonal relationships, play and leisure time, coping skills) and motor skills (gross and fine motor). This measure was selected because it is a reliable and valid diagnostic tool. American Guidance Service, Inc. (Circle Pines, MN 55014) publishes this test.

The *Bayley Scales of Infant Development, Infant Behavior Record (IBR)* uses descriptive rating scales of behavior characteristics to assess children up to 30 months of age. The scale focuses on interpersonal and affective domains, motivational variables, and a child's interest in specific modes of sensory experience. Specifically, the *IBR* yields ratings in Social Orientation, Cooperativeness, Fearfulness, Tension, General Emotional Tone, Object Orientation, Goal Directedness, Attention Span, Endurance, Activity, Reactivity, Sensory Areas of Interest Displayed, Energy and Coordination for Age, Judgment of Test, Unusual or Deviant Behavior, and General Evaluation of Child. The *IBR* provides a convenient form for recording qualitative observations and evaluations and concludes with a general evaluation of the child's overall performance. An examiner completes the *IBR* immediately after administering the Mental and Motor Scales. It is completed by indicating the one statement that best describes the child's behavior. Additional space is provided for the examiner's comments about the child, which can broaden the base upon which to make clinical judgments.

The *Child Behavior Checklist* (Achenbach 1989) was designed to obtain standardized data on children's competencies and problems, as reported by their parents or parent-surrogates. It may be administered by an interviewer or self-administered. Assessments of changes over time or following treatment may be obtained by readministering the instrument. Separate interview forms are available for 2- to 3-, and 4- to 5-year-olds. The authors recently added several helpful changes, including instructions for obtaining uniform demographics, and room for open-ended items concerning illnesses and handicaps, the informant's concerns, and the best thing about the child. Using clinical cutoff points, problems in the areas of social withdrawal, depression, sleep problems, somatic problems, aggression, and destructiveness may be ascertained. The Child Behavior Checklist is available by writing to Thomas M. Achenbach, University of Vermont, Department of Psychiatry, 1 South Prospect Street, Burlington, VT 05401.

Communication. A number of assessments are available to evaluate communication skills. Only a few that are widely used are reviewed here. Because of the complexities of assessing communication in children with severe motor dysfunction, the reader is referred to the book, *Neurodevelopmental Strategies for Managing Communication Disorders in Children with Severe Motor Dysfunction* (Langley and Lombardino 1991).

The *Sequenced Inventory of Communication Development* (Hedrick, Prather, and Tobin 1975) is a standardized instrument designed for children whose chronological age is between four months and four years, or for those who are developmentally delayed. Designed to measure receptive and expressive language, the test takes between 30 and 75 minutes to administer, depending upon the age of the child. By combining direct observation of the child with parental input, the test yields information about a wide range of skills. Interobserver agreement was .96 and test-retest reliability was .93. Correlations with scores on the Peabody Picture Vocabulary Test were .75 to .80.

The *Receptive-Expressive Emergent Language Scale (REEL)* (Bzoch and League 1970), is a test designed to provide developmental information about the child's communicative behavior. The instrument assesses prelinguistic skills in infants between one month and three years of age. Through parent reports, a receptive and expressive communication age score is obtained.

The *Test for Auditory Comprehension of Language (TACL)*, (Carrow-Woolfolk 1973) is a reliable instrument that measures receptive language in the areas of vocabulary, morphology, and syntax. It was designed for children between three and six years of age, and requires no verbal responses, relying solely on the child's choice of a picture in response to an examiner's verbal stimuli. (It is, therefore, also usable with children or adults with language disorders, severe hearing impairments, mental retardation or aphasia.) Information obtained from the *TACL* results can provide the clinician with information about a child's understanding of vocabulary, grammar, and syntax.

The *Peabody Picture Vocabulary Test, Revised Edition (PPVT-R)* (Dunn and Dunn 1981), is a well-standardized instrument designed primarily to measure receptive vocabulary. (This instrument was not selected for obtaining measure of cognitive functioning because it measures only one facet of general intelligence, namely, vocabulary.) Inasmuch as only a pointing response is required, it is appropriately used with nonspeaking and nonreading clients. It takes approximately 10 to 20 minutes to administer and score the test and it is recommended for individuals between $2^1/2$ and 40 years old. Reliability falls in the satisfactory range (.70s). It also correlates quite strongly with other instruments testing vocabulary.

Play behaviors. Play behaviors should be assessed in several different contexts. To observe the child's varying play skills, interaction abilities, and the parent's capacity to facilitate the child's play skills, ask the parent to play with the child in several different play situations. Several play scales are available; however, many more are not published or readily available. One play-based assessment that is available is the *Transdisciplinary Play-Based Assessment* (Linder 1990). This naturalistic, functional assessment is developmental in nature and is based upon the observations of the transdisciplinary team, consisting of both parents and professionals. The assessment is designed to identify service needs, to develop intervention plans, and to evaluate progress in children who are functioning at a level between six months and six years. Observation guidelines are presented in cognitive, social-emotional, communication and language, and sensorimotor development. These guidelines may be used to observe various play and interaction skills, in addition to other areas of development. The assessment is available through Paul H. Brookes Publishing Co., Baltimore, MD.

Summary

This chapter reviews a number of strategies for assessment of emotion regulation, communication, play, and interactions. Because children with neuromotor dysfunction frequently have limited skills in these areas, it is important to address these areas in assessment and treatment. When standardized assessments are not appropriate for a child because of the severity of the handicap, use naturalistic observations through play-based assessments.

7.

SENSORY PROCESSING

Overview of Sensory Processing

From a developmental standpoint, the infant learns to detect and interpret information from the senses during the first two years of life. The various sensory systems (i.e., tactile, vestibular, and vision), through strong neural connections with the motor system, create maps of the body and interpret the environment in a way the body can process usefully. In essence, the sensory and motor "maps" are linked with one another in the brain. Multiple maps are created so that the child can conceptualize or visualize himself in many different positions doing many different activities. Thus, the "maps" of self and environment interact to allow for the development of adaptive motor responses, motor planning and motor control, coordination of the two body sides, postural stability, body scheme, self-image, balance, and eye-hand coordination.

It has been hypothesized that adaptive responses impose organization on the central nervous system (CNS) by providing sensory feedback about a goal-directed event (Ayres 1975, 1985). The ability to process and organize sensory information goes beyond the motor system, however. Sensory processing is also essential in the regulation of arousal and attention (Kopp 1982), and in emotional and behavioral control (Greenspan and Porges 1984).

In this chapter, the somatosensory, vestibular, and proprioceptive systems are described. The presenting symptoms of children with sensory processing difficulties for each system are discussed, with emphasis on the problems of children with neuromuscular dysfunction. Motor planning deficits are also described. Since it is often difficult to administer standardized sensory assessments (i.e., *Test of Sensory Functions in Infants; DeGangi-Berk Test of Sensory Integration*) to children with neuromuscular dysfunction, a set of qualitative observations that can be used to measure change in a child's sensory responses are presented also. These measures may be used for baseline and retest measures.

The Somatosensory System

The somatosensory system is a primal sensory system that responds to various touch stimuli on the surface of the skin. It is a predominate sensory system at birth and remains critical throughout life as a major source of information for the central nervous system. An infant's first movements are made in response to tactile input (eg: rooting reflex, palmar grasp reflex, stepping response). These early sensorimotor experiences are "stored" in the brain (e.g., thalamus, parietal lobe), where they are used to create effective motor responses (Ayres 1985).

The sense of touch involves the ability to receive and interpret sensation and stimuli through contact with the skin. The child's responses to tactile input give us a great deal of information about the degree of tactile integration present in the child's nervous system. Problems in the tactile system not only affect motor and reflex development, but also tactile perception, motor planning, and emotional stability (Ayres 1972).

The tactile system serves two functions: protection and discrimination. The tactile protective system plays an important role in survival by lending a general tactile awareness of the environment. Temperature changes of the skin, light touch, and general contact with the skin can activate this function. This system is concerned with general aspects of tactile sensation, particularly the qualitative nature of external stimuli and, consequently, is linked with emotional responses to touch. It acts as a protective mechanism to the central nervous system by giving warning if an outward stimulus is too close for safety. In the newborn child, this protective reaction predominates until the baby becomes accustomed to being touched and learns to discriminate which tactile experiences are dangerous and which are enjoyable. Children who are unable to tolerate light touch and are highly sensitive to tactile experiences such as standing next to another child, wearing a long sleeved shirt, or even sitting on a chair are termed "tactually defensive." Often hyperactivity is associated with the problem.

A second important function of the tactile system is discrimination, which involves responses to deep touch-pressure, touch combined with motion, and the precise localization of touch. The development of tactile discrimination (e.g., the ability to differentiate various textures, contours, and forms by feel) plays an important role in adaptive motor behaviors, particularly in the initiation and planning of movement (Ayres 1972) and exploration of the environment. If the tactile discriminative system is not functioning properly, the child has difficulty in orienting toward and organizing tactile input in time and space in a meaningful manner. This explains why there are many children with poor tactile discrimination who cannot sequence skills such as dressing. Another important function of the tactile discriminative system is to give us emotional tone or emotional stability while engaged in tactile stimulation activities. For instance, the mother who burrows her face on her baby's tummy in a game of touch should elicit smiling and laughter from her baby. The infant or child with poor tactile discrimination may avert its gaze, pull away from the contact, or even cry.

A child who does not actively manipulate an object or interact with the environment adaptively reflects one of the most common problems related to poor tactile discrimination. Since hand skills involve many discrete manipulations of an object, fine motor skills are often compromised in the child with poor tactile discrimination. If a child is unable to manipulate an object because of muscle tone abnormalities, the problem is compounded. If the discriminative system is not functioning properly, the child will not be able to organize tactile input in time and space in a meaningful manner. This process is important for the proper development of social interactions and emotional behaviors.

For normal development to occur, the protective and discriminative systems must balance. When the CNS malfunctions, as we observe in children who are learning disabled or have cerebral palsy, the nervous system tends to regress to a developmentally earlier response that has greater survival value. In these children, the protective system is over-aroused. They experience as unpleasant or threatening the kind of tactile stimulation that most people would consider pleasurable. If the child rejects tactile experiences, he will avoid using his body and hands to explore his world. Important motor milestones—such as crawling, or extensive manipulation of objects—may be bypassed. The child may avoid being held, or may not tolerate close proximity with others due to an intolerance to touch. These behaviors have important implications for emotional development.

Somatosensory Dysfunction

The tactile dysfunctions that are most commonly observed in children are tactile defensiveness and tactile hyposensitivities. The tactile problems of the child with neuromuscular dysfunction (e.g., cerebral palsy) have received little attention in the literature. Reactions to somatosensory stimuli can range from overresponsivity to underresponsivity. Overresponsivity is commonly characterized by feelings of discomfort and physical withdrawal from certain types of tactile stimuli. Ayres has described this as tactile defensiveness (1972, 1979, 1985).

Sensitivities to touch may be environmental (e.g., fleeing from contact of furniture or equipment; discomfort from the touch of clothing), other-initiated (e.g., withdrawal from mother hugging child; avoidance of being in groups of children), or self-initiated (e.g., avoidance of touching textured objects). The child may respond aggressively by hitting or kicking, or by physically retreating (e.g., hiding under furniture). Emotional responses, including hostility, are not uncommon.

Tactile defensiveness. Tactile defensiveness is the severe sensitivity to being touched. Usually it involves an adverse reaction to initiating touch as well. Touch experiences that are normally perceived as pleasant are viewed as noxious. The child with tactile defensiveness will express feelings of discomfort and a desire to escape from the situation involving touch. The symptoms are much worse in situations where touch is forced upon the child rather than initiated by the child. The child responds by attempting to remove himself from the situation and will state, "I hate this game. It hurts," or "It tickles." The child may pull away from being touched, run away from the adult, hit or kick aggressively, or hide under furniture. Even if the child is touched slightly, he may exclaim, "Don't push me!" or "Watch where you're going!" Anxiety, discomfort, a need to withdraw, and hostility are common behavioral manifestations of tactile defensiveness (Ayres 1972; Ayres and Tickle 1980; Bauer 1977).

The phenomenon of tactile defensiveness is characteristic of some children with learning disorders and has been correlated with hyperactivity and distractibility. It has also been documented in autistic children (Ayres and Tickle 1980). Inadequate cortical inhibition of sensory processing and poor regulation in the reticular activating system has been speculated to cause symptoms of increased activity level, sleep/wake disturbances, tactile defensiveness, or withdrawal from sensory stimulation (Fisher, Murray, and Bundy 1989; Montagu 1978).

Tactile defensiveness occurs when the lemniscal system doesn't inhibit the spinothalamic system and the reticular activating system becomes stimulated as a result. The reticular activating system is very sensitive to adrenaline, which in turn causes such behaviors as: an increased activity level, distractibility, and a restless or fidgety nature. This alteration in the reticular activating system lowers the individual's threshold of sensitivity, causing over-sensitivities to smell and sound. In some children, there may be bizarre emotional reactions to stimuli. For instance, one infant would begin to cry uncontrollably at the sight of rain on a windshield, possibly because of the feeling associated with rain falling on herself.

Tactile hyposensitivities. Decreased tactile awareness—or a hyperreactivity to touch—is seen less often than tactile defensiveness. Children experiencing hyporeactivity to touch do not experience touch unless the experience is very intense. Such a child may laugh and actually appear to enjoy a firm pat on the buttocks when being disciplined. A characteristic of the child who is hyporeactive to touch is a lack of reaction to pain. The child acts as though no pain is felt. Some children may bite themselves very hard, actually breaking the skin without reacting. Children with diminished tactile awareness are very slow in initiating movement and exploring objects by feel. The child with this problem is in essence suffering from a type of sensory deprivation. Very often children with either tactile defensiveness or tactile hyperreactivity will exhibit a lag in motor development because of their inefficient use of touch in exploring objects.

Somatosensory problems in children with neuromuscular dysfunction. Children with neuromuscular dysfunction may display tactile defensiveness by fisting their hands, arching away from the stimulus, or standing on their toes. Tactile defensiveness in the child with neuromuscular dysfunction may be primary or secondary in nature. For instance, movement limitations cause the child with spasticity to have difficulty weight bearing and weight shifting over body surfaces. This in turn results in tactile deprivation to certain body parts or surfaces. It may be difficult for this child to engage in normal patterns of play that routinely provide sensory input (e.g., touching hand to foot in play, or exploring textured objects in play). In addition, the typical postures assumed by hypertonicity (e.g., shoulder elevation and retraction) may shelter certain body parts from normal tactile stimulation. Children with hypotonicity may exhibit tactile defensiveness in the same way that the hypertonic child does, because environmental exploration is difficult.

Children can also display hyposensitivity to somatosensory input. These children typically do not seem to experience touch unless the stimulus is very intense; it is as if their thresholds for noticing or reacting to stimuli are very high. Often these children do not seem to experience pain, are slow to initiate movement for tactile exploration, and therefore also suffer from a type of sensory deprivation.

It is common for these children to seek touch-pressure input. Some self-abusive behaviors may be interpreted as a means to trigger very high pressure thresholds (e.g., biting, head banging). Frequently, children with this difficulty have low muscle tone, perhaps related to poor sensory support for movement experiences. Their patterns of stability and movement reflect this condition. For instance, one may see the child sitting half-on and half-off of a chair or sitting with an arm caught under the body with no apparent discomfort. These children may hit or bite themselves when frustrated with no evidence of pain, or laugh when they receive a firm pat on the buttocks when disciplined. They usually love rough handling and seem to need intense and prolonged contact before they respond appropriately. Hypertonic children may exhibit tactile hyposensitivities as well. For instance, the child may display an abnormal craving for intense or very familiar tactile experiences. For example, the child might enjoy touching a rough, bristly hairbrush, but pull away from a soft, furry puppet. It is important to note that the same child may exhibit elements of both tactile hyper- and hypo-reactivity to tactile experiences (e.g., crave deep pressure contact on hands, but show an aversion to light touch or certain textures on palms).

The Vestibular System

The vestibular system, like the tactile system, is a predominate sensory system at birth that has a major impact on emotional stability. Vestibular system structures include the labyrinths of the inner ear, which are sensitive to positional changes of the head in space. The eyes also provide input to the vestibular system, maintaining the plane of vision for balance and detecting whether the body or another object is moving in space. Because it helps the infant orient himself in space and initiate exploratory and adaptive movements, the vestibular system, along with the tactile system, is particularly critical for the development of basic functions in the young infant (Naunton 1975).

It affects the development of body posture, muscle tone, ocular-motor control, reflex integration, and equilibrium reactions. These vestibular-based functions have a strong impact on the development of motor skills, visual-spatial and language abilities, hand dominance, and motor planning (Clark 1985; DeQuiros 1976; Keshner and Cohen 1989; Ottenbacher 1982).

An important function of the vestibular system is to provide a sense of gravitational security to the body as it moves. It has been described as playing an important role in the development of emotional stability as well as balance, postural mechanisms, and spatial perception. A child without adequate vestibular function may be insecure in his body movements and fearful of movement in space (particularly in leaving his feet off the floor). As a result, this insecurity is likely to foster emotional instability in the child as well.

Vestibular Dysfunction

Vestibular dysfunction has been documented in a variety of learning and emotional disorders. Most notably it has been observed in autistic children and schizophrenic adults. Some autistic children crave spinning, while others prefer to look at spinning objects such as fans and wheels. The autistic child may climb to precarious heights and positions, showing remarkable ease with balance. Schizophrenic adults, on the other hand, have been described as experiencing motion sickness, resisting movement activities, and holding their bodies in a stooped, flexed posture. It seems then that a disturbance in the vestibular system can take several forms.

Two common problems associated with vestibular dysfunction, gravitational insecurity and hyporeactivity to movement in space, are described below.

Gravitational insecurity. Ayres (1972) has described the phenomenon of gravitational insecurity, which is seen in some learning and emotionally disturbed children. The gravitationally insecure child will demonstrate extreme fearfulness of moving in space and will have a strong preference for upright, close-to-ground body positions. Postural or gravitational security seems to play an important role in the development of emotional stability, as well as in balance, postural mechanisms, and spatial perception.

Children who have a low tolerance for movement (hypersensitivity to movement) are usually overwhelmed by powerful movement stimuli such as spinning, frequent changes in direction and speed, or unusual body positions (e.g., inverted). Typically they are fearful about leaving the earth's surface and thus are called gravitationally insecure (Ayres 1979). Often they will display considerable autonomic responses (dizziness, nausea) during and after any type of vestibular stimulation. Children with this problem typically have a strong preference for upright positions, 'lock' the body in rigid postures to avoid movement stimulation and resist participation in activities with these components. Not only are they fearful of body movement in space, but they also resist any change in their body position, which they may perceive as threatening. Their postural adjustments tend to be very rigid, and they are most fearful of inverted body positions. Children with hypertonicity may be hypersensitive to movement; this may be due to lack of experience with the input received or an inability to develop a repertoire of acceptable movement patterns in response to the input.

Children with gravitational insecurity need to be introduced to new movement through a slow, gradual approach. Because they lack confidence in their movement through space, children with gravitational insecurity tend to be very emotionally unstable. They frequently display a fearfulness of new situations, rigidity, and a resistance to change.

Hyporeactivity to movement in space. Children who are hyporeactive to movement usually crave movement experiences and yet do not seem to profit from them. Because the tolerance is high, one often sees less autonomic responses associated with movement (e.g., dizziness). There are some children who appear to be hyporeactive in their excessive craving for movement in space who do display autonomic responses (i.e., nystagmus), but who do not know how to interpret these responses. They seem to lack an internal barometer that helps gauge and register the perception of movement. Often these children are very emotionally unstable and tend to overstimulate themselves because they lack this internal regulatory feedback mechanism. One may see explosive movement quality, poor judgment in starting and stopping movement activities, or difficulty with transitional movements. The child with low muscle tone may not be able to move against gravity easily enough to stimulate the vestibular system in a variety of movement planes; poverty of movement provides fewer opportunities for developing vestibular output for postural control.

The Proprioceptive System

The proprioceptive system develops through weight bearing and movement against gravity. This sense is critical in the maturation of reflexes, particularly the righting and equilibrium reactions, in perception of body position and movement in space and against gravity, and in providing postural security and stability as the child moves throughout the environment. Visual feedback is important in monitoring posture and movement; visual/proprioceptive integration is critical to the refinement of spatial concepts and body percept (Fisher and Bundy 1989; Matthews 1988).

Proprioceptive Dysfunction

Proprioceptive dysfunction is frequently seen in conjunction with somatosensory or vestibular dysfunction; this is probably because of the brain's multiple shared processing regions. Behaviors that are commonly associated with poor proprioceptive processing include over- or undershot limb movements, locking of joints for stability, poor placement of the extremities for weight bearing (e.g., wide base support pattern, weight bearing on dorsum of hand), poor muscle co-contraction and holding against gravity, poor righting and equilibrium reactions, and difficulty grading and modulating movement. Insecurity in moving in space is also associated with poor vestibular-proprioceptive processing and involves extreme fearfulness in leaving the earth's surface, fear of heights, and emotional insecurity during movement activities.

Motor Planning Disorders

Developmental dyspraxia, also known as a *motor planning disorder,* is a sensory processing deficit that typically has its base in either the tactile or vestibular system. The problem lies not so much in the processing of sensory input or the ability to produce the movement skill, but in the intermediary process of planning the movement. The child with dyspraxia has significant problems in planning and carrying out goal-directed movement, skilled, or non-habitual motor tasks. The dyspraxic child is often vulnerable to distraction as a result because he lacks the internal organization to focus his behavior.

There are several distinct types of motor planning problems. They include postural dyspraxia, sequencing praxis, oral and verbal praxis, constructional and graphic praxis, and dyspraxia of symbolic use of objects. *Postural praxis* is demonstrated when the child is unable to plan and imitate large body movements and meaningless postures. A *sequencing praxis* occurs when the child has difficulty making transitions from one motor action to another and in sequencing movements (e.g., thumb-finger sequencing). *Oral praxis* is the inability to produce oral movements on verbal command or in imitation. Children with oral praxis usually have poor speech articulation. *Constructional praxis* is the inability to create and assemble three-dimensional structures (e.g., block bridge). *Graphic praxis* involves the inability to plan and execute drawings. (Since there is a component of visual-spatial perception in drawing and construction, graphic and constructional praxis are not based solely on a motor planning deficit.) *Symbolic praxis* involves the inability to use objects symbolically (Ayres 1985; Cermak 1985).

Some of the common symptoms of the child with dyspraxia are delays in dressing, and delays in fine and gross motor skills involving imitation, sequenced movements (i.e., lacing, skipping), and construction (i.e., building from a block model). Poor accuracy of movement is observed in the dyspraxic child, and skilled hand movements, such as handwriting, are typically very difficult for the child to execute. Their movement quality may be described as explosive, with poor judgment of force, speed, and aim. Speech articulation may also be poor since this is a planned, skilled motor activity. Non-habitual tasks are most difficult for dyspraxic children; therefore, they prefer routines and strongly resist changes. Transitions from one activity to the next may cause behavioral upset.

Initiation of new movement sequences or new organized plans of behavior are difficult. For instance, the child may not be able to tell you what he plans to do because he lacks an internal plan. As a result, one may see the dyspraxic child as either very disruptive and aggressive, particularly when there is no external structure to organize the child, or as very passive, preferring the repetition of certain favorite activities, and resisting new and different tasks. One may observe tantrums, aggressive behavior, poor play skills with peers, frustration, and a strong resistance to change. Some children become very controlling and manipulative because of their inability to control and impact their environment. Needless to say, poor self-concept is a major problem of the dyspraxic child.

Assessment of Sensory Processing Problems in Children

The instruments that may be used for testing sensory processing and reactivity are:
- for infants, the *Test of Sensory Functions in Infants (TSFI)* (DeGangi and Greenspan 1988)
- for preschoolers, the *DeGangi-Berk Test of Sensory Integration (TSI)* (DeGangi and Berk 1983) and the *Touch Inventory for Preschoolers* (Royeen 1987)

Each test is described in the next section.

Standardized measures. The *Test of Sensory Functions in Infants (TSFI)* (DeGangi and Greenspan 1988) is a 24-item test developed to measure sensory processing and reactivity in infants. It focuses on evaluation of responses to tactile deep-pressure, visual-tactile integration, adaptive motor skills, ocular motor control, and reactivity to vestibular stimulation. The instrument has been validated on a sample of 288 normally developing, 27 developmentally delayed, and 27 difficult-temperament infants from 4 to 18 months. Psychometric studies of the instrument reveal that:

—the items and subtests validly measure the domain of sensory functioning in infants;

—the total test scores can be used reliably and validly for screening decisions, particularly for 7- to 18-month-old infants;

—the five subtests can be used reliably and validly for guiding clinical decisions for infants with delays or difficult temperament at 10 to 18 months of age (DeGangi, Berk, and Greenspan 1988).

Interobserver reliability ranged from .88 to .99 for the subtests. The total test and test-retest reliability was .81 overall. In addition, decision consistency reliability ranged from 81 to 96% for the total test scores. Western Psychological Services (12031 Wilshire Boulevard, Los Angeles, Calif. 90025) publishes the test.

The *DeGangi-Berk Test of Sensory Integration (TSI)* (DeGangi and Berk 1983) may be used with preschool age subjects with mild motor handicaps. The criterion-referenced test was designed to measure overall sensory integration in 3- to 5-year-old children with delays in sensory, motor, and perceptual skills, or for children suspected of being at risk for learning problems. Its focus is primarily on the vestibular-based functions and includes subtests measuring postural control, bilateral motor integration, and reflex integration. It is a useful test for screening and diagnosing children with sensory integrative dysfunction. Also, the test may be useful in delineating areas in need of therapeutic intervention. Interobserver reliability were .80 to .88 for the subtests and total test, except for the Reflex Integration subtest, which was .66. Test-retest reliability was .85 to .96 and decision-consistency reliability was .83 to 100%. Western Psychological Services (12031 Wilshire Boulevard, Los Angeles, Calif. 90025) publishes the test.

The *Touch Inventory for Preschoolers (TIP)* (Royeen 1987) measures tactile defensiveness in preschoolers. It is a rating scale with 46 questions that is completed by the parents. The questionnaire has been validated on a sample of preschoolers and is useful in delineating children who have sensitivities to touch.

Formal testing of sensory integrative functioning may be conducted using the *Sensory Integration and Praxis Tests (SIPT)* (Ayres 1989). This test, designed for children at 4 years, 0 months through 8 years, 11 months, includes measures of: vestibular, proprioceptive, and somatosensory processing; visual-perceptual/motor integration; integration of the two body sides; and praxis. The praxis tests measure postural imitation; motor planning in response to a verbal request; motor sequencing ability; imitation of oral movements; graphic reproduction; and three-dimensional block construction. Because the *SIPT* requires the child to engage in complex motor actions, it is not recommended for children with neuromotor dysfunction.

Clinical observations. The following list of clinical observations may be used to observe whether a child has sensory dysfunction. These observations may be used during the baseline, then repeated to measure progress after intervention. Tables 7.1 to 7.3 present the observations for somatosensory and vestibular dysfunction and motor control and planning problems.

TABLE 7.1
Clinical Observations of Somatosensory Dysfunction

Tactile hypersensitivities:

1. Dislikes being touched or cuddled by others: pulls away from being held, arches, grimaces; cries or whines.

2. Distressed when people are near, even when they are not touching (i.e., standing nearby, sitting in a circle).

3. Avoids touching certain textures. Hates getting hands messy (i.e., fingerpaints, paste, sand).

4. Likes firm touch best (i.e., seeks firm hugs from others).

5. Prefers touch from familiar people.

6. Dislikes having face or hair washed. Especially dislikes having a haircut.

7. Prefers long sleeves and pants, even in warm weather. OR prefers as little clothing as possible, even when it's cool.

8. Touches everything in sight.

9. Bumps hard into other people or objects.

10. Withdraws from being near others, particularly groups.

11. May hit, kick, or bite others, and is aggressive in play.

12. Has a strong preference for certain food textures (e.g., only firm and crunchy, or only soft).

13. Dislikes being dressed or undressed.

14. Resists being placed in certain positions (e.g., stomach, back).

Tactile hyposensitivities:

1. Seems unaware of touch unless it is very intense.

2. Does not react to pain (e.g., shots, scrapes).

3. Bites or hits self.

4. Likes to hang by arms or feet off of furniture or people.

5. Unaware of messiness around mouth or nose.

Poor tactile discrimination (for children over two years):

1. Has difficulty with fine motor tasks (e.g., holding pencil, buttoning).

2. Always looks at hands when they are manipulating objects.

3. Uses mouth to explore objects.

TABLE 7.2
Clinical Observations of Vestibular Dysfunction

Vestibular hypersensitivities:

1. Is easily overwhelmed by movement (e.g., carsick).

2. Has strong fear of falling and of heights.

3. Does not enjoy playground equipment and avoids roughhousing play.

4. Is anxious when feet leave ground.

5. Dislikes having head upside down.

6. Is slow in movements such as getting onto therapy bench or walking on an uneven surface.

7. Is slow in learning to walk up or down stairs and relies on railing longer than other children same age (pertains to children with mild motor delays).

Under-responsiveness to movement:

1. Craves movement and does not feel dizziness when other children do.

2. Likes to climb to high, precarious places.

3. Has no sense of limits or controls.

4. Is in constant movement, rocking, running about.

TABLE 7.3
Clinical Observations of Motor Control and Motor Planning Problems

Motor control:

1. Frequently breaks toys—cannot seem to judge how hard or soft to press when handling toys.

2. Trips over obstacles or bumps into them.

3. Falls frequently (after 18 months).

4. Assumes slumped body posture when sitting or standing.

5. Leans head on hand or arm.

6. Prefers to lie down than sit, or to sit rather than stand.

7. Has a loose grip on objects such as a pencil, scissors, or spoon, *or* grip is too tight on objects.

8. Fatigues easily during physical activities.

9. Is loose jointed and floppy; may sit with legs in a W.

10. Has difficulty manipulating small objects, particularly fasteners.

11. Eats in a sloppy manner.

TABLE 7.3 (continued)
Clinical Observations of Motor Control and Motor Planning Problems

Motor planning:

1. Fear of trying new motor activities. Likes things to be the same and predictable (i.e., routine).

2. Difficulty making transitions from one activity to next.

3. Must be prepared in advance several times before change is introduced.

4. Cannot plan sequences in activities; needs structure from an adult.

5. Is easily frustrated.

6. Is very controlling of activities.

7. Has difficulty playing with peers.

8. Is aggressive or destructive in play.

9. Throws temper tantrums easily.

10. Did not crawl before starting to walk.

11. Has difficulty with dressing and sequenced motor actions (e.g., skipping, scissor cutting, buttoning).

Assessment Techniques to Quantify Changes in Sensory Processing

1. Select two or three goals for sensory processing that the parent and therapist agree are treatment priorities. These might include:

   a. initiates exploration of textured toys when several appealing toys are presented to the child (duration of time spent exploring; frequency of touching textured objects during a set period of time)

   b. tolerates being placed on back for diapering, bathing, and other daily care tasks (number of times tolerates back during day versus number of times cried, whined, or fussed)

   c. can be dressed or bathed without fussing or crying (number of times was happy and content during dressing or bathing versus frequency of times child was fussy, whining, etc.)

   d. tolerates being held by therapist or parent for therapy exercises (number of minutes that therapist or parent can hold child to do therapy activities)

   e. initiates movement into backward or lateral directions without showing fear response (when presented with an interesting set of toys behind the body, number of times child spontaneously reaches behind body or out to sides within a set period of time)

   f. presence of self-abusive behaviors (e.g, biting hand)

   g. presence of temper tantrums over course of day

Some of these behaviors may be noted by the parent using a daily log. Others may be observed during a therapy session.

Define exactly how you will measure the behavior each time that you are observing it. For example, you may select a bin filled with dried beans within which are buried several of the child's favorite toys. You may set out the bin and within a three-minute observation, time how long the child touches the beans and textured toys, or use the number of objects retrieved from the bin as your criteria. Develop a procedure for motivating the child to do the task, and describe it. Consider the following points when developing your measures.

1. Define behavior being observed.
2. Describe criteria for performance in simple terms.
3. Describe stimuli used to elicit behavior (toys, materials, any procedures).
4. Determine the duration for the observation before and after treatment. It should only be a few minutes.
5. Decide how a daily log might be used to record behaviors.
6. Determine how the child's responses will be coded (i.e., frequency, duration).

Summary

This section outlines various assessment procedures that may be useful in documenting somatosensory, vestibular, and proprioceptive dysfunction, and motor planning problems in infants and children. A combination of formal and informal assessment procedures are recommended, particularly in light of the fact that the sensory tests described were not validated on children with severe motor dysfunction. The section describing methods to quantify day-to-day changes in sensory processing should be useful in developing observations that are meaningful and that impact functional performance.

8.

ATTENTION AND AROUSAL

Attention, alertness, and arousal are important for basic survival. They contribute to the ability to filter out irrelevant information, to tune into important elements in the environment, to process new information for learning, and to engage in purposeful activity. The construct of attention is highly multi-faceted and involves components of arousal and alerting, habituation and interest in novelty, capacity to sustain effort, selection and screening of stimuli, and motivation and persistence in attention (Davies and Parasuraman 1984). This process operates within the context of what the individual already knows about the world and the types of stimuli, tasks, and events that are encountered.

Why Is It Important to Measure Attention?

The process of sustained attention, particularly the ability to differentiate novel and familiar stimuli, has been identified as important in the development of later cognition (Bornstein and Sigman 1986; Fagan 1982; Rose and Wallace 1985; Ruff 1986). Sustained attention is defined as the ability to direct and focus cognitive activity on specific stimuli. It is reflected by how long an infant will engage in cognitive schemes involving the stimulus (e.g., visual inspection, manipulation), once attention has been drawn toward the task or event. Kopp (1982) proposed a theory of self-initiated regulation of behavior that extended the definition of sustained attention to include the ability to initiate, maintain, and cease activities in relation to task and situational demands. The capacity to self-initiate goal-directed activity while sustaining attention in the absence of external monitors from others is central to information processing.

How Does Attention Impact Function?

In order for an individual to attain functional competence, it becomes crucial that attention to ongoing routine sensory stimulation be passive and involuntary. When an individual is constantly attending to things like the feel of clothing on his body or the constant drone of a fan, there is little reserve for active voluntary attention to more meaningful environmental events or internal thoughts. Likewise, when a child is constantly attuned to shifts in muscle tone or extraneous involuntary movements, it becomes difficult to sustain attention. When a person is actively engaged in voluntary attention, functional purposeful activity and learning can occur.

Without the ability to sustain attention, the person would not be able to process information and develop cognition. The ability to attend selectively helps the individual select or focus on one type of information to the exclusion of others. Motivation and persistence also contribute.

Attention Deficits: What Are They?

One of the core symptoms of behavior disorders such as hyperactivity, learning disorders, and mental retardation is a deficit in attention. Attention deficit disorder has been described as a constellation of symptoms that includes distractibility; poor concentration and lack of persistence; poor self-monitoring; disorganization; and impulsivity. Prospective studies of attention deficit disorder have confirmed that children in this population are at high risk for academic underachievement and behavioral difficulties (Carey and McDermitt 1980; Rutter 1982). Persistent inattention in early childhood has also been associated with poor achievement in reading and mathematics in the second grade (Palfrey et al. 1985).

There are different types of attentional deficits. Children diagnosed as having an attentional deficit do not always fit into well-defined categories with uniform characteristics. The etiologies of attentional disorders are many and often nebulous. Many researchers contend that the etiology is a function of neurologic dysfunction.

Impaired sensory registration. Impaired sensory registration is a common problem affecting attentional abilities. A pattern of overarousal is seen when there is difficulty filtering extraneous information. Accompanying this picture are problems with orienting to irrelevant stimuli, distractibility, excessive motor activity, and a decreased attention span. In contrast, a pattern of underarousal may be manifested in two ways: as a high activity level associated with stimulus-gathering behaviors; or as a low activity level, with difficulty orienting and acting upon novel stimuli. Often parents and professionals view a high activity level as a symptom of *over*arousal (e.g., the child fleeing from stimulation), but it can also mean that the child is underaroused and is seeking stimulation. Often the child is not processing the sensory information properly, but sometimes the child seeks the sensory inputs that are not useful to further learning (i.e., objects that can be spun or twirled).

Impaired information processing. Impaired information processing may be associated with attentional deficits. Inabilities to accurately identify stimuli or to detect all the sensory qualities may be the result of an inability to sustain attention. The attentional deficit may mean the individual does not orient appropriately to novel stimuli, has difficulty attaching meaning to input, and does not organize adaptive responses for efficient performance. This inability to redirect attention to salient stimuli may result in an apparent behavioral perseveration. Concurrent with these problems may be deficits in information storage and retrieval necessary for learning. In addition, dyspraxia (e.g., disorder in planning and organizing adaptive motor responses) is often observed as well.

A deficiency in behavioral inhibition. This condition is a component of the attentional disorder. Behavioral inhibition is necessary for optimal sustained attention and appears to have a parallel in the autonomic nervous system (e.g., the lowering and stabilizing of autonomic activity) (Porges 1984).

Difficulties modifying actions and adapting to environmental demands. These problems accompany an attentional deficit. Behavioral responses are often stereotypic and perseverative in nature. Often the child is bound by previously learned and explicitly taught behaviors. The ultimate impact of the attentional disorder is on development of communication, perception, learning, and social-emotional skills.

Assessment Strategies for Attention

One way to assess attention is through administration of a standardized cognitive test. Two cognitive tests that may be used for this purpose are the *Bayley Scales of Infant Development* (Bayley 1969) and the *McCarthy Scales of Children's Abilities* (McCarthy 1972). After administering the *Bayley Scales,* the *Infant Behavior Record* form may be completed to describe the child's response to testing, which includes various attentional measures. If the child is older than 2½ years, a variety of attentional observations may be made following administration of the *McCarthy Scales.*

The *Bayley Scales* and *McCarthy Scales* are described below, followed by a variety of clinical observations that may be noted during administration of the *McCarthy Scales.*

The *Bayley Scales of Infant Development* is a reliable and convenient indicator of child development for infants and toddlers. One part of the scales, The Mental Development Index (MDI), measures cognitive and perceptual abilities. It was designed to assess sensory-perceptual acuities, discriminations, and ability to respond to acquisitions of "object constancy" and memory, learning, and problem-solving ability; vocalizations and the beginnings of verbal communication; and early evidence of an infant's ability to form generalizations and classifications, which is the basis of abstract thinking. The results of the Mental Development Scale are expressed as a standard score, called the Mental Development Index. The Psychological Corporation (555 Academic Court, San Antonio, TX 78204-0952) publishes the test.

The *McCarthy Scales of Children's Abilities* (McCarthy 1972) is a test of general cognition and motor abilities for children from 2½ to 8½ years. It is standardized and has been shown to be reliable and valid. The test scores yield a profile in five domains (Verbal, Perceptual-Performance, Quantitative, Memory, and Motor) as well as a general cognitive index. The Psychological Corporation (555 Academic Court, San Antonio, TX 78204-0952) publishes the test.

The *Bayley Scales of Infant Development: Infant Behavior Record (IBR)* consists of descriptive rating scales of behavior characteristics of children up to 30 months old. The scale focuses on interpersonal and affective domains; motivational variables; and a child's interest in specific modes of sensory experience. Specifically, the *IBR* yields ratings in Social Orientation, Cooperativeness, Fearfulness, Tension, General Emotional Tone, Object Orientation, Goal Directedness, Attention Span, Endurance, Activity, Reactivity, Sensory Areas of Interest Displayed, Energy and Coordination for Age, Judgment of Test, Unusual or Deviant Behavior, and General Evaluation of Child. The *IBR* provides a convenient form of recording qualitative observations and evaluations and concludes with a general evaluation of the child's overall performance. An examiner completes the *IBR* immediately after having administered the Mental and Motor Scales. It is completed by indicating the one statement that best describes the child's behavior. Additional space is provided for an examiner's comments, which can broaden the base upon which to make clinical judgments about a child.

Clinical Observations of Attention

In addition to structured observations of attention, a checklist is provided in table 8.1 for use in documenting attentional problems.

Day-to-day observations to document changes in attentional abilities. Therapist and parent observational measures used to document changes in attention should be geared specifically toward the type of attentional problem observed in the child. Some examples are presented here of how these may be observed by a therapist.

1. **Child will sit at the table for perceptual or fine motor activities without being distracted by environmental stimuli.**

    a. How long did child sit at the table for fine manipulative or other table top tasks during the session?

    0-1 minute ___

    2-5 minutes ___

    6-10 minutes ___

    More than 10 minutes ___

TABLE 8.1
Clinical Observations of Attention

1. Is vulnerable to distractions (e.g., sights or sounds); is distracted at least three times during testing by environmental stimuli.

2. Has a high activity level; is constantly running about and is unable to sit still for an activity. Attempts to leave table three or more times during testing. May stand up for parts of table top testing. May need several breaks from testing.

3. Plays only briefly with toy before wanting a new activity.

4. Is impulsive in handling materials, needing three or more reminders to wait before touching.

5. Tunes out from activity; is difficult to reengage. Processing of directions is slow; urging is needed to elicit response.

6. Can't shift focus easily from one object or another after playing for long period of time.

7. Gives up easily. Is frustrated and needs urging to persist.

8. Prefers only easy tasks.

9. Wanders aimlessly, without focused exploration.

10. Depends upon an adult to focus attention during play activities.

11. Becomes excited when confronted by crowded, bustling settings such as a crowded supermarket, restaurant.

      b. Was child distracted by sounds, sights, etc.? Y ___ N ___

Did child redirect himself to task
on his own?   Y ___ N ___

How often was the child distracted?

At least once/minute: ___

Several times in 5 minutes: ___

Only a few times in 15 minutes: ___

2. Was sitting at table for focused perceptual or fine motor activities self-initiated by child?   Y ___ N ___

By therapist?   Y ___ N ___

3. Did child resist structure imposed by therapist?   Y ___ N ___

4. Was child able to transition from therapy to the waiting room after treatment without behavioral resistance or disorganization (i.e., increased activity level)?   Y ___ N ___

5. **Was child able to persist on difficult motor tasks involving organization and planning?**

   a. Did child give up quickly?   Y ___ N ___

   b. Did child need only encouragement to persist?   Y ___ N ___

   c. Did child visually attend to a gross motor sequence demonstrated by therapist?   Y ___ N ___

   d. Did child imitate a simple gross motor task?

      1-step (i.e., jump on trampoline)   Y ___ N ___

      2-step (i.e., jump, then throw ball)   Y ___ N ___

      3-step (i.e., in obstacle course)   Y ___ N ___

   e. Was verbal cuing needed during sequence?   Y ___ N ___

Because sensory stimulation or inhibitory activities may impact the child's capacity to attend, the child's response to tactile or movement activities may be observed each session. Observations may include the following:

1. **Did child seek heavy deep-pressure tactile activities during session?**   Y ___ N ___

   For how much of session did child want this input?

   Briefly ___ 3-5 min. ___ 6-10 min. ___ 11-15 min. ___

   Most of session ___

2. **What was child's activity level like after tactile stimulation activities?**

   Aggressive ___ Fragmented attention ___

   Focused attention on one activity ___

   Better motor planning ___ Other:

Summary

This chapter presents a variety of methods for observing attentional responses during functional activities. Because the construct of attention is very complex, it is important to delineate the various ways that the child is able to attend, screen out irrelevant stimuli, process information, and control impulses. Not only should attention be measured, but it should be addressed in the treatment process, since the capacity to focus attention during purposeful activities is key to learning and generalization of skills.

Appendix A

CASE DESCRIPTIONS

Appendix A presents six cases that show how the assessment procedures described in this manual are applied. Each case includes pertinent history, the pre-test observations, parent concerns, the daily observation log completed by the parents and therapist, a description of the therapy program, gains made from therapy, and a summary of overall progress as perceived by the family. Each child received eight weeks of neurodevelopmental treatment provided by either an occupational or physical therapist.

Note: To protect privacy, names and other non-essential identifying details have been changed for the subjects appearing in the case studies.

Case Description 1: John

John is an adorable 2-year-old of Asian-Caucasian descent. He has received physical therapy from six months of age, when he was initially diagnosed as being hypotonic with developmental delays in cognition, language, and motor skills. At 13 months, he began participation in a school-based educational and therapeutic program, where he receives daily intervention. John's parents have been very involved in his therapy program, integrating suggestions from the teachers and therapists into various daily living and play activities.

Pertinent History

John was delivered by Caesarian section at 30 weeks' gestation, with a birth weight of 3 pounds. Apgars were 5 and 8. During the pregnancy, his mother developed diabetes and had premature labor two weeks prior to delivery. John experienced apnea, bradycardia, pulmonary artery branch stenosis, and hyperbilirubinemia, for which he was hospitalized three months. At 15 months of age, John experienced febrile seizures. He has pneumonia, asthma, ear infections, and severe allergies.

Developmental History

John's social-emotional skills are his strength, an area that has been age appropriate. In general, he has experienced developmental lags in all areas, with the mildest lags in cognition (3- to 4-month delay). At 24 months, gross motor skills fell at approximately the 9- to 12-month level, fine motor skills were at the 13-month level, and speech and language skills at the 13- to 15-month level.

Primary Presenting Problems
(Pre-Test Observations)

The primary problems that were identified as needs during the assessment are presented in table A.1.

TABLE A.1
Primary Presenting Problems: John

---

1. Weakness in controlling graded flexion/extension of the lower extremities, with inability to lower self from stand to squat in order to pick up toys from the floor and to hold a bear position. Back-kneeing with weight on heels is observable in standing. When moving out of standing, the legs buckle and collapse due to underlying low tonus and muscle weakness.

---

2. Lack of trunk rotation in various developmental positions affecting functional skills such as getting in and out of child-sized chair, or holding a side-sitting position while reaching upward and across body for toy.

---

3. Weak thoracic extension in developmental positions. When sitting on bench with feet supported, John cannot reach upward with both hands to grasp large object. Thoracic spine is rounded, with compensatory neck hyperextension.

---

4. Difficulty isolating individual finger movements such as pointing with index finger at objects. The thumb is inactive in grasp patterns such as holding a string.

---

5. Tonus in the trunk is low, with postural fixations affecting anti-gravity postural control. When standing at furniture, John leans his body against any available surface.

Parents' Concerns

The primary areas expressed by the parents as areas of need included the following:

1. Feeding skills, including the ability to self-feed with a spoon and to drink from a cup.
2. Skills that will enable John to explore the environment and play with toys, such as opening a door by turning a handle or knob, or pulling a string to obtain a toy.
3. Fine motor skills involving grasp and release (e.g., stacking blocks) and tool use (e.g., crayon).
4. Gross motor skills, with emphasis on developing independent standing.

Measures Completed by Therapist

The measures completed by the therapist after each therapy session are presented in table A.2.

Log Completed by Parents

John's parents recorded specific observations in a log two or three times a week. The behaviors they looked for are presented in table A.3.

TABLE A.2
Measures Completed by Therapist: John

1. Develop graded flexion/extension of lower extremities in standing.
   a. Lowers self slowly to squat position to pick up toys on floor. Y N
   b. Holds bear position while reaching for toys between legs
      and out to body sides Y N
      Requires: Minimal assist _____
      Maximal assist _____
      No assist _____

2. Improve trunk rotation in various developmental positions.
   a. Gets in and out of child-sized chair using trunk rotation. Y N
   b. Holds side-sitting position while reaching up and across
      body diagonally. Y N

3. Improve thoracic extension in developmental positions.
   a. While sitting on bench with feet supported, John reaches
      upward with both hands to grasp large object. Thoracic spine
      is extended without neck hyperextension. Y N
   b. John reaches behind him to obtain toy while sitting on bench. Y N

4. Improve isolated finger use.
   a. Points with index finger at objects or to gesture. Y N
   b. Uses thumb actively in grasp pattern (i.e., pulls string toy,
      or pushes with thumb in opposition pattern to activate toy) Y N

5. Improve tonus in trunk.
   a. Stands at furniture without leaning into it. Y N
   b. Pushes cart while walking without leaning trunk on handles. Y N

TABLE A.3
Log Completed by Parents: John

1. Feeds self with spoon without help: Y N

   Feeds self with spoon with minimal help: Y N

2. Stirs spoon in cup: Y N

3. Puts cup down with small spill (i.e., no more than one
   tablespoon lost): Y N

   Puts cup down with no spill: Y N

4. Opens door, turning handle or knob: Y N

5. Pulls string toy: Y N

6. Stacks two-cube tower: Y N

7. Scribbles with crayon: Y N

8. Stands alone: Y N

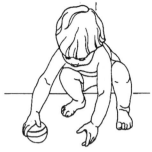

Figure A.1. Stimulate squat to standing position by encouraging child to reach in various ways for a toy.

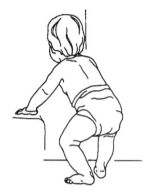

Figure A.2. Encourage child to move from standing to squat positions to pick up objects from the floor.

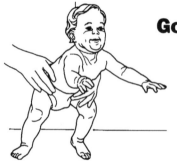

Figure A.3. Maintain leg separation and give intermittent support to quadriceps to prevent child from collapsing to floor when moving into squat position.

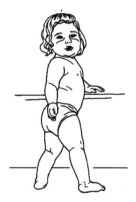

Figure A.4. Encourage child to reach behind self for objects while standing against a toy kitchen sink or other support.

Description of the Therapy Program

Individualized physical therapy was provided twice a week in 30-minute sessions by a physical therapist using a neurodevelopmental treatment approach. The therapist had more than 10 years' experience in working with children with motor impairments and in the application of neurodevelopmental treatment. Therapy was provided in a therapy room within a school setting, although consultation to the classroom teacher and parent were considered essential to the therapy program and occurred on an ongoing basis. Suggestions were made to the parents and teachers to enhance carryover of skills. The emphasis in therapy was on direct physical handling, parent and teacher education, home and classroom programming, and positioning for skill development in the classroom and home settings. The therapist used a variety of handling techniques and tools, including mobile equipment and stationary surfaces (such as benches). At the onset of the therapy program, the therapist needed to guide John's movement using key points on the trunk, pelvis, and lower extremities. However, as John progressed in his capacity to hold body postures against gravity, in functional skill development, and in his motivation to move, the therapist could rely more heavily upon positioning a toy or activity in certain ways to encourage specific movement patterns. Toys and activities were used to motivate John to move or to engage in functional activities.

Goals and Techniques

Goal 1: Improve lower-extremity strength in graded flexion/extension activities.

Techniques:

a. Stimulate squat to standing while reaching between legs, or to either right or left of legs, for toy on floor (figure A.1).

b. Practice squatting as a play position.

c. Move from standing to squat to pick up objects on floor (figure A.2).

d. Provide intermittent pressure to gluteals to encourage hip extension in standing (figure A.3). Maintain leg separation and intermittent support to quadriceps to prevent collapse to floor when moving into squat.

Goal 2: Improve trunk rotation in various developmental positions.

Techniques:

a. Reach for objects across body midline.

b. Standing at toy kitchen sink, reach behind self for objects (figure A.4).

c. Straddle legs over small bench and reach behind body for toys.

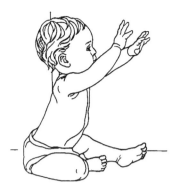

Figure A.5. Stimulate child to reach overhead for toy while child is in sitting position.

Goal 3: Improve thoracic extension in developmental positions.

Techniques:

    a. Stimulate reaching overhead for toys in sitting, half-kneeling, and kneeling (figure A.5).

    b. Encourage ball throwing overhead.

    c. Practice lifting lightweight blocks overhead with both upper extremities.

    d. Practice standing and placing balls in large bin.

Goal 4: Improve simultaneous activation of trunk extensors and flexors and weight shifts during standing and walking activities.

Techniques:

    a. Climb over bench, step in and out of cart, and step over other obstacles.

    b. Push cart and cruise along wall (figure A.6).

    c. Creep up and down ramp.

    d. Place balls in bins while standing.

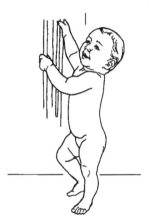

Figure A.6. Cruising along a wall stimulates weight shifts and coactivation of the child's trunk.

Improvements in Skills from Pre- to Post-Assessments

1. Lower extremity skills

   Pre-assessment: Creeps on one knee and one foot instead of reciprocal creeping pattern; unable to cruise by furniture; depends upon furniture for support in standing, leaning abdominals onto surface (figure A.7); stands with help from an adult with feet planted in a wide base of support.

   Post-assessment: Reciprocal creeping pattern; cruises by furniture and wall surface; climbs over obstacles; stands at furniture without leaning abdominals onto surface; stands with support with normal base of support.

2. Transitional movements and trunk rotation

   Pre-assessment: Lack of trunk rotation in transitional movements, with use of highly symmetrical movement patterns; when required to turn to reach for toy, turns entire body and hyperextends neck to look behind or to side.

   Post-assessment: Uses trunk rotation to reach behind body and to cross the body midline without neck hyperextension pattern; transitional movements show trunk rotation; development of new skills, such as sitting down into child-sized chair from standing, using trunk rotation.

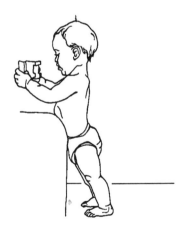

Figure A.7. This child depends upon furniture for support in standing.

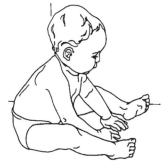

Figure A.8. This child shows thoracic rounding.

3. Upper extremity skills

Pre-assessment: Uses elevated shoulders and neck hyperextension for overhead reach; unable to reach overhead to full range due to thoracic rounding (figure A.8); difficulty holding weighted toy in space.

Post-assessment: Reaches overhead with full thoracic extension and without neck hyperextension; holds weighted toy in space while playing with it.

Overall Gains

Significant progress was found overall in skills that were observed by the therapist as well as those observed by the parents. The 16 therapy sessions were divided into four equal periods and the data were inspected for the presence or absence of skill completion. Likewise, the number of parent observations were divided into quarters and the results analyzed for evidence of improvement over time. They are presented in table A.4.

TABLE A.4
Improvements Observed by Therapist: John

	1st quarter	2nd quarter	3rd quarter	4th quarter
Skill completion	31	34	39	40
Unable to complete skill	9	6	1	0

Improvements observed by the parents over time are presented in table A.5.

TABLE A.5
Improvements Observed by Parents: John

	1st quarter	2nd quarter	3rd quarter	4th quarter
Skill completion	11	13	15	20
Unable to complete skill	29	27	25	20

Gains in specific skills observed by therapist. John demonstrated significant improvements in nine of ten skills observed by the therapist. The number of times that John was able to perform a skill during or immediately after a therapy session was tallied across the 16 sessions. The results are presented in table A.6.

TABLE A.6
Gains Made in Skills Observed by Therapist: John

Skill	Number of Times Completed
1. Squatting in play	16/16
2. Holding bear position with minimal to no assistance	11/16
3. Trunk rotation in getting in and out of chair	15/16
4. Side-sitting with upward reach	16/16
5. Sit with thoracic extension and upward reach	15/16
6. Reach behind back with thoracic extension	14/16
7. Points with index finger	14/16
8. Thumb active in grasp	16/16
9. Stands without leaning on furniture	16/16
10. Pushes cart	15/16

Gains made in specific skills observed by parents. Significant changes in specific skills observed by the parents were found in two of eight skills measured. The results are presented in table A.7. Many of the skills observed by the parents emerged near the end of the eight-week therapy program.

TABLE A.7
Gains Made in Skills Observed by Parents: John

Skill	Number of Times Completed
1. Feeding with some help	24/25
2. Stirs with spoon	4/25
3. Puts cup down without spill	22/25
4. Opens door	1/25
5. Pulls string toy	0/25
6. Stacks 2-cube tower	6/25
7. Scribbles	10/25
8. Stands alone	2/25

Description of Progress Obtained in Parent Interview

John's mother was interviewed to determine the ways in which she feels her son has improved during the eight-week therapy program that were not captured by the daily observation measures.

Motor. John is squatting in play, standing more of the time, and cruising by furniture with confidence. His feet look more active instead of being so flat. He doesn't lean against furniture when standing or cruising. His movement looks more automatic instead of jerky. He has more finger control and will hold small objects longer. He does more with his hands, using his fingertips more instead of only his palm.

Dressing. He can pull his shirt off and on and will weight shift to put on his pants. He is fussing more with dressing because he knows what he wants to do.

Communication. John is more verbal and more purposeful in his gestures. His intention is clearer so that the parents don't need to guess what he wants.

Cognition. John has shown tremendous cognitive growth over the two months. He has become very interested and motivated to explore his environment as he developed more motor control. He is able to follow directions.

Play. John's play has become more purposeful and creative with more variety in how he manipulates toys.

Emotion. John is less dependent on his parents. Separation anxiety is observed less as he has become more adventurous in seeking new experiences.

Summary

At the conclusion of the therapy program, John at 26 months had demonstrated significant progress in lower extremity control, squatting, standing, cruising, trunk rotation, feeding skills, and isolated finger movements and refined pincer grasp. Postural tone had improved so that John did not need to rely upon equipment or table surfaces to hold him up when standing. This was evidenced as well in the therapist's ability to change from controlling the trunk as a key point in therapy to simply encouraging movement patterns by using toys and activities while guiding movement in a more minimal fashion. Significant progress was noted in overall gains observed both by the therapist and the parents. Additionally there was significant progress in specific skills that were observed during pre- and post-test measures and behaviors observed by the therapist and parents over time. The results are very encouraging in the treatment of this 2-year-old child with hypotonia and developmental lags.

Case Description 2: Nina

Nina is a 13-month-old child of black-Caucasian descent with severe feeding problems. She was referred for occupational therapy at nine months by a developmental follow-up clinic because of feeding problems that included vomiting, possible reflux, and an inability to suck from a bottle. She was also diagnosed as having spastic quadriplegia. She had recently begun the county school parent-education program where she receives specialized therapy services twice a week. The parents, particularly the father, have been very involved in Nina's therapy program, which is primarily directed toward feeding and motor concerns. Because of her extreme feeding problems, extensive hospitalization following a traumatic birth, and other family life events that occurred at the time of the referral, the parents were experiencing a high degree of stress. Nina began treatment in the research project at 11 months.

Pertinent History

Nina was born prematurely, at $3^1/2$ months, at a birth weight of 1 lb., 1 oz. Neonatal complications included respiratory distress syndrome, necrotizing enterocolitis, retinopathy of prematurity, apnea, and bradycardia. Nina was on a ventilator for one month and remained on an apnea monitor through ten months. Apnea spells occurred during both sleep and feeding. She has had a history of reflux, and at 12 months, midway through the therapy program, she received a gastrostomy because of severe failure to thrive.

Developmental History

Nina has significant developmental delays in all areas. At nine months ($5^1/2$ months corrected age for prematurity), she performed at the 4.4-month level in motor and cognitive skills. Nina has been diagnosed as having a significant neurosensory hearing loss. She is deaf in her left ear, with partial hearing on the right. She has increased muscle tone with persistence of primitive reflexes. She can sit with maximal support, prop in prone briefly, and reach with her right hand for faces and objects.

Feeding history. Feeding is a major problem. Nina takes as long as two hours to consume four ounces. During bottle feeding, Nina will arch, turn her head away, bat at the bottle, and will hold the formula in her mouth without swallowing. Because Nina has difficulties with bottle feeding, her parents have resorted to using a very large opening in the nipple or spoon feeding liquids into her mouth. Often Nina will vomit after eating. Her mother reported that Nina often does not show hunger and can go 12 hours without eating. Despite Nina's eating difficulties, she is showing good weight gain and continues to show growth on her growth curve. She weighs 13 lb., 13 oz., and is 24 inches long.

Primary Presenting Problems (Pre-test Observations)

The primary problems that were identified during the assessment prior to treatment in the research project are presented in table A.8.

TABLE A.8
Primary Presenting Problems: Nina

1. Increased extensor hypertonicity, which is observable during rolling from stomach to side and when held in sitting or at the shoulder; inability to flex neck and trunk in supine; partial optical righting reactions in prone and with lateral displacements only.

2. Strong extensor tone in the legs when supine or held upright with standing on toes.

3. Hand fisting with difficulty bringing the hands to the midline, and persistence of the asymmetrical tonic neck reflex.

4. Difficulty grasping and holding toys, particularly with the left hand.

5. Significant hypersensitivities to touch around the lips and in the mouth; gagging of the tongue and arching of the head are associated with touch on the tongue.

6. Hyperactive gag reflex with vomiting due to reflux.

7. Lack of lip closure, with inability to initiate a suck-swallow or latch onto a nipple; difficulty coordinating breathing while sucking and swallowing.

8. Hypersensitivities to touch resulting in total inhibition of arousal (e.g., drops off to sleep when touch is sustained in holding contact).

Parents' Concerns

The primary areas expressed by the parents as areas of need included the following:

1. Development of motor skills, including crawling and sitting

2. Awareness and use of left arm and leg

3. Decrease extensor tone

4. Tolerate touch to the mouth

5. Improve hand-eye coordination

Measures Completed by Therapist

The measures completed by the therapist following each therapy session are presented in table A.9.

TABLE A.9
Measures Completed by Therapist: Nina

1.	Normalization of hypersensitivities to touch around lips and in mouth	
	a. Tolerates touch around lips:	Y N
	b. Tolerates touch in mouth (without gagging, crying, vomiting):	Y N
2.	Inhibition of gag reflex	
	a. Nipple of bottle can be placed in mouth without gag:	Y N
	b. Spoon can be placed firmly on tongue without gag:	Y N
3.	Improve lip closure	
	a. Closes lips around nipple, maintaining a good seal:	Y N
4.	Improve suck and swallow	
	a. Sucks continuously on bottle during feeding:	Y N
	Duration of time that sucks continuously: _____	
	b. Amount of fluid ingested:	Y N
	Duration of feeding: _____	
	Amount ingested: _____	
	c. Evidence of vomiting during session:	Y N
	Frequency: _____	
5.	Inhibition of neck and trunk hyperextension	
	a. Neck hyperextension observed when held in supported sitting:	Y N
	b. Rolls with hyperextension of trunk:	Y N
	c. Brings hands to knees or feet in supine while tucking neck:	Y N
6.	Improve hand function	
	a. Hands are open most of time:	Y N
	b. Holds toy and shakes or manipulates it:	Y N
	c. Hands hold bottle:	Y N
	d. Brings hands to mouth:	Y N
	e. Hands are in midline during play:	Y N

Log Completed by Parents

A log of observations was completed by the parents two or three times a week during the course of the therapy program. The behaviors they looked for are presented in table A.10 (see page 78).

TABLE A.10
Log Completed by Parents: Nina

1.	Tolerates touch around lips:	Y	N
2.	Tolerates touch in mouth (without gagging, crying, vomiting):	Y	N
3.	Nipple of bottle can be placed in mouth without gag:	Y	N
4.	Spoon can be placed firmly on tongue without gag:	Y	N
5.	Closes lips around nipple without losing milk:	Y	N
6.	Length of time taken to drink bottle: _____ Amount ingested: _____		
7.	Vomiting during feeding?	Y	N
	Frequency: _____		
	Vomiting after feeding?	Y	N
8.	Holds toy and shakes or manipulates it:	Y	N
9.	Hands hold bottle:	Y	N
10.	Brings hands to mouth:	Y	N
11.	Healthy and feeling good that day:	Y	N
12.	Practiced home program exercises:	Y	N
13.	Any new concerns?		

Description of the Therapy Program

Nina was treated twice a week in one-hour sessions over the course of eight weeks by an occupational therapist trained in neuro-developmental treatment. The therapist had more than 10 years' experience in working with children with motor impairments and in the application of neurodevelopmental treatment. Therapy was provided primarily in the home, although a few sessions were held at an outpatient clinic. The emphasis in therapy was on direct physical handling, parent education and home programming, and positioning for feeding and play in the home. The therapist used a variety of handling techniques and tools, including handling on her lap, mobile equipment and positioning equipment (e.g., feeder chair). Key points used in handling varied according to task demands and position but were primarily on the trunk, shoulders, and pelvis, except when work was directed toward feeding. Throughout the handling program, toys and activities were used to motivate Nina to move or engage in functional tasks. Simple materials—such as easy-to-grasp toys—were employed, or visually interesting targets (e.g., mirrors, pictures).

Goals and Techniques

The goals and therapy techniques that were used in Nina's therapy program are described in detail below.

Goal 1: Decrease extensor hypertonicity in the neck, trunk, and extremities, and improve anti-gravity flexion.

Techniques:

a. Pelvic elevation in supine to inhibit extensor tonus in pelvis with neck flexed. Facilitate hands to midline, and hands to knees or feet (figure A.9).

b. Sitting while activating weight shifts laterally and in anterior-posterior direction.

c. In sidelying, stimulate midline play with both hands while keeping neck laterally flexed against gravity and elongation of one body side.

Goal 2: Improve hand use, specifically grasping of toys and hands to midline while inhibiting asymmetrical tonic neck reflex.

Techniques:

a. In supine flexion position, stabilization of shoulders provided so arms may be lifted up against gravity to reach for toy in midline (figure A.10).

b. In sidelying, stimulate hands to midline in handling easy-to-grasp, medium-sized objects (figure A.11).

c. While prone on therapy ball, use of weight shifts in lateral and anterior-posterior directions to inhibit fisting of hands and to facilitate grasping of objects in prone, propping with arms in forward position.

d. Stimulate left-hand awareness by weight bearing and weight shifts onto left arm in prone (i.e., stroking with interesting, textured toy) (figure A.12).

e. Propping in prone over a small therapy roll to enhance weight bearing and weight shifting on flexed elbows during play (figure A.13).

Goal 3: Decrease hypersensitivities to touch around the lips and in the mouth; inhibit hyperactive gag, and improve lip closure and suck-swallow.

Techniques:

a. Position for feeding using tumble form feeder chair to inhibit arching.

b. Stimulation using NUK® toothbrush by helping Nina guide toothbrush in her mouth by herself.

c. Introduce spoon, using firm pressure on tongue to inhibit gag and facilitate coordinated swallow.

d. Using firm touch-pressure, touch on cheeks and lips in playful game prior to feeding.

e. Using cup, stimulate lip closure around cup's edge by providing support under lower lip; introduce small amount of fluid at a time.

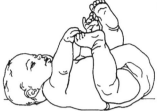

Figure A.9. Facilitate child's hands to midline, and hands to knees or feet to help decrease extensor hypertonicity in the neck, trunk, and extremities.

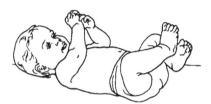

Figure A.10. Shoulders are stabilized in a supine flexion position so that child may lift arms against gravity to reach for toy in midline.

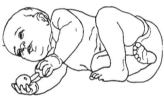

Figure A.11. Hands are stimulated to midline in sidelying when handling easy-to-grasp, medium-sized objects.

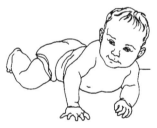

Figure A.12. Weight shifts in lateral and anterior-posterior directions facilitates propping with arms in forward position.

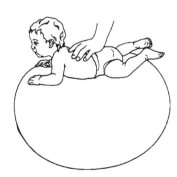

Figure A.13. Propping on hands and elbows in prone on a therapy ball enhances weight bearing and weight shifting.

Improvements in Skills from Pre- to Post-Assessments

1. Optical righting reactions

   Pre-assessment: Partial in prone and lateral directions.

   Post-assessment: Full adjustment in prone and lateral; sluggish adjustment in supine.

2. Sitting equilibriums

   Pre-assessment: Absent.

   Post-assessment: Partial trunk and full head response in lateral directions; full head in anterior and posterior planes.

3. Protective reactions in sitting

   Pre-assessment: Absent.

   Post-assessment: Weight on fisted hand in lateral and forward displacements.

3. Pull to sit

   Pre-assessment: Head hangs but slight assist with shoulders and neck present.

   Post-assessment: Head initiates.

4. Tonus in trunk and upper extremities

   Pre-assessment: Moderate to high resistance, with fisting of hands; stiffness in trunk with hyperextension.

   Post-assessment: Mild resistance with open hands; intermittent tendency to arch trunk, with persistent stiffness in symmetrical postures.

5. Tonus in lower extremities

   Pre-assessment: Lower extremities extend in supine with plantar flexion; stand on toes in supported standing.

   Post-assessment: Legs can be freely abducted in supine with no resistance; continual tightness in hamstrings with straight leg raise; stands on toes in supported standing.

6. Persistence of primitive reflexes

   Pre-assessment: Presence of ATNR, positive supporting, palmar and plantar grasp reflexes, and Moro, with full response for all of these.

   Post-assessment: Minimal postural response on ATNR to both sides; palmar grasp faded; minimal plantar grasp and partial abduction on Moro only observed; positive supporting remains present.

7. Functional motor skills

Pre-assessment: Sits with maximal support at trunk; rolls to side from supine with hyperextension; props on forearms with arms under body.

Post-assessment: Sits independently but with intermittent arching of trunk and shoulder retraction; rolls from supine to prone; supports weight in prone extension pattern.

8. Hand skills

Pre-assessment: Hands fisted most of time; no use of left hand.

Post-assessment: Grasps using radial digital grasp in both hands; reaches for objects with either hand; scoops pellets with either hand; rotates wrist, right hand only.

9. Sensory processing

Pre-assessment: Hypersensitive to touch on face and body; hypersensitive to movement-in-space activities.

Post-assessment: Normal responses to tactile deep pressure on body, mild sensitivities to textured objects; hypersensitive to movement in inverted planes.

10. Feeding

Pre-assessment: Two hours to feed four ounces; gagging with nipple or spoon; vomiting; holds food in mouth.

Post-assessment: Accepts food from spoon and will feed 10 spoonfuls of pureed food at a time; accepts water from cup; swallows without facilitation, imitates speech sounds during feeding; vomiting no longer occurs; one hour to feed six ounces.

Overall Gains Made in Therapy

Significant progress was found overall in the change in skills that were observed by the treating therapist as well as the parents. The 16 therapy sessions were divided into four equal periods; the data were inspected for presence or absence of skill completion. The results are presented in table A.11.

TABLE A.11
Improvements Observed by Therapist: Nina

	1st quarter	2nd quarter	3rd quarter	4th quarter
Skill completion	23	34	37	35
Unable to complete skill	21	10	7	9

These results show significant improvement over the 16 treatment sessions.

Likewise, the number of parent observations were divided into quarters. A few of the parent measures were discarded because of their lack of applicability, including those that involved the use of the bottle, which was discarded after the gastrostomy. The results of the parent measures are presented in table A.12.

TABLE A.12
Improvements Observed by Parents: Nina

	1st quarter	2nd quarter	3rd quarter	4th quarter
Skill completion	19	24	30	31
Unable to complete skill	16	11	5	4

These results show significant improvement over the 16 treatment sessions.

Gains made in specific skills observed by therapist. Nina demonstrated significant improvements in eight of 11 behaviors. The behaviors involving the bottle were discarded since these were not observed continuously over the 16 treatment sessions. Likewise, the food intake measure and time required to eat were not valid measures over time because of the insertion of the gastrostomy midway through the treatment regime. The number of times that Nina was able to perform a skill during or immediately after a therapy session were tallied across the 16 sessions. Table A.13 presents the findings.

TABLE A.13
Gains Made in Skills Observed by Therapist: Nina

Skill	Number of Times Completed
1. No hypersensitivity to touch on lips	16/16
2. No hypersensitivity to touch in mouth	14/16
3. No gagging with spoon	13/16
4. No vomiting	15/16
5. No neck hyperextension in supported sitting	10/16
6. Rolls without neck hyperextension	2/16
7. Reaches for feet or knees	7/16
8. Hands open	13/16
9. Holds toy in hands	16/16
10. Brings hand to mouth	14/16
11. Brings hands to midline	13/16

Gains made in specific skills observed by parents. Significant changes in specific skills observed by the parents were found for six of seven measures. The results are presented in table A.14.

TABLE A.14
Gains Made in Skills Observed by Parents: Nina

Skill	Number of Times Completed
1. Tolerates touch around lips	18/20
2. Tolerates touch in mouth	15/20
3. Spoon can be placed in mouth without gag	13/20
4. Closes lips on nipple or spoon	15/20
5. No vomiting	16/20
6. Holds toys	16/20
7. Brings hands to mouth	18/20

Gains made during the parent observations corresponded with gains observed by the therapist, with the exception of placing the spoon in the mouth without gagging. This seemed largely attributable to the parents' consistent capacity to position Nina in a chair for feeding. Apparently the feeding chair was on loan to the family and was not available for all sessions. For other sessions, they positioned her in a walker, infant seat, or held her in their arms, with variable success.

Description of Progress
Obtained in Parent Interview

Nina's father was interviewed to determine the ways in which he feels that Nina improved in the eight-week therapy program that were not captured by the daily observation measures.

Health. When the therapy program was initiated, Nina's parents were concerned about whether she would live or die because her feeding problem was so severe. Now they are concerned about whether she will walk. The gastrostomy was important in stabilizing Nina medically. She has had an enormous weight gain and is now too fat and happy—weighing 23 lbs. at 14 months.

Feeding. Although Nina continues to resist feeding, she is much easier to feed. She is no longer sensitive to touch in her mouth and does not gag anymore.

Motor. Nina's ability to move, and her drive to move, have improved dramatically over the past two months. She is able to sit for up to five minutes at a time, and she now uses her left hand to hold rattles. Her tone problem seems mainly in her left arm.

Communication. Nina is making more sounds and expressing herself more during play and everyday activities.

Summary

At the conclusion of the therapy program, Nina was 13 months old. She had demonstrated significant progress in reflex maturation (e.g., righting and equilibrium reactions with decrease in primitive reflex activity), postural tone (decrease in stiffness in extremities and trunk), motor skill development (sitting, rolling, and prone propping), functional grasp patterns, particularly in the use of the left hand, decreased sensitivities to touch in the mouth and body, and improved feeding from the spoon and cup. She swallows now without vomiting or gagging. This case example demonstrates how gains can be documented in pre- and post-assessment measures, and through regular observations made by the therapist and parents. Overall gains were made across the areas measured, as well as in specific skills. Nina will continue to require therapy and educational interventions to address her ongoing needs; however, her progress from the program is highly encouraging.

Case Description 3: Gus

Gus is a 13-month-old Caucasian boy. He was referred for developmental evaluation at 11 months by his pediatrician because of generalized hypotonia. Comprehensive testing was conducted in a hospital-based developmental evaluation clinic. Testing revealed significant delays in motor and cognitive skills. It was recommended that Gus receive intensive physical and occupational therapy, in addition to being referred to an early intervention program in the county school system. Gus had just begun physical therapy when he participated in the NDT research project.

Pertinent History

Gus was born full-term at a birth weight of 6 lbs., 11 oz. Seven months into the pregnancy, his mother experienced a flu virus, with a temperature of 102°. At delivery, apgar scores were 5 at one minute and 9 at five minutes. Gus was described as blue initially and received oxygen in the delivery room. He developed jaundice that resolved without phototherapy.

At 10 weeks, Gus sustained a serious head injury when he fell from his mother's arms, requiring significant suturing of a laceration on his forehead. A CT scan of the brain and X-rays of the spine were normal. A genetic evaluation was conducted because of minor dysmorphic facial features and ulnar drift of the fingers. Genetic abnormalities were ruled out.

In addition to the referral for developmental evaluation, Gus was seen by an ophthalmologist because of esotropia of the left eye, for which patching was recommended.

Developmental History

When tested at 11 months, Gus functioned at the seven-month level in motor skills and at the $7^1/_2$-month level in cognitive skills. He could sit when placed, but often fell backwards, and he could not move in and out of sitting. His highest skill was making stepping movements.

When put on his stomach, he would cry. Grasping objects was difficult for Gus because of ulnar deviation of the wrists and hyperextension of the fingers. An unusual posturing of the hands was observed also. Gus was alert and interested in sound production but was noticed to be sensitive to loud noises. Generalized low muscle tone was observed, with immature righting and equilibrium reactions.

Primary Presenting Problems (Pre-Test Observations)

The primary problems identified during the assessment, prior to treatment in the research project, are presented in table A.15.

TABLE A.15
Primary Presenting Problems: Gus

1. Poor postural stability and control in anti-gravity positions, including difficulty pushing up onto hands and knees, commando-crawling, or moving out of prone or supine against gravity.

2. Reliance on postural fixation in the neck and trunk, with a preference for symmetrical postures with poor trunk rotation. As a result, mobility skills were delayed, particularly transitional movements such as rolling from supine to prone.

3. Difficulty utilizing left body side, affecting functional use of the upper extremity, trunk rotation, and weight bearing on that side as in side sitting on the left.

4. Poor midline organization in bimanual tasks.

5. Lack of refined thumb-fingertip grasp patterns and wrist rotation.

6. Difficulty initiating, problem-solving, and planning new motor actions.

Parents' Concerns

The primary concerns expressed by the parents included:
1. Ability to drink from a bottle or cup independently

2. Ability to self-feed finger foods

3. Development of mobility skills, including creeping, rolling, and pushing up to a quadruped position

4. Ability to pull to sit or assume sitting independently

5. Capacity to fall and stay asleep

6. Tolerance for being placed on his stomach without fussing or crying

Of these issues, the parents were most concerned about Gus' capacity to fall and stay asleep. The parents experienced feelings of great stress as a result of many sleepless nights.

Measures Completed by Therapist

Measures completed by the therapist after each therapy session are presented in table A.16.

TABLE A.16
Measures Completed by Therapist: Gus

1. Improve trunk rotation in sitting.
   a. Reaches laterally to body side with left hand to reach for toy: Y   N
   b. Rotates trunk toward left body side with right hand or shoulder, crossing midline to reach for toy: Y   N
   c. Assumes side-sitting position on left side: Y   N
   d. Holds side-sitting position for one minute or longer on right side: Y   N

2. Improve mobility skills in low-to-ground positions.
   a. Rolls over from supine to prone with encouragement of interesting toy: Y   N
   b. Rolls toward right body side: Y   N
   c. Pivots in $1/4$ to $1/2$ turn in prone: Y   N
   d. Pushes up onto hands and knees and rocks: Y   N
   e. Moves forward on floor in prone position: Y   N
   f. When left by himself on mat on back for three minutes, what does he do:
   Lies there?   Y   N
   Rolls over?   Y   N

3. Develop midline hand skills.
   a. Holds large object (e.g., ball) with two hands in midline: Y   N
   b. Holds large object and raises it overhead in play using two hands: Y   N
   c. Holds weighted toy with two hands for one minute or longer: Y   N

4. Develop hand skills.
   a. Holds small objects with inferior pincer: Y   N
   b. Holds small objects with refined pincer: Y   N
   c. Points with index finger: Y   N
   d. Rotates wrist so that toy is in vertical alignment (i.e., peg, small people toy):   Y   N

Log Completed by Parents

The parents made entries into a log two to three times a week during the course of the therapy program. The behaviors they looked for are presented in table A.17 (see page 88).

TABLE A.17
Log Completed by Parents: Gus

1. Holds bottle by self with two hands:	Y	N
For how long? _____		
2. When left on floor on his back for several minutes, what does he do?		
Is content on back:	Y	N
Rolls over:	Y	N
Cries and fusses:	Y	N
3. Moves about on belly on floor when encouraged to move:	Y	N
4. Picks up piece of dry cereal (such as oat circle) with refined pinch:	Y	N
5. Falls asleep without needing to be breast fed:	Y	N
6. Wakes in night and needs help to fall back to sleep or becomes distressed and cries:	Y	N
7. Is healthy and feeling good on day of observation:	Y	N

Description of the Therapy Program

Gus received physical therapy twice a week in a private physical therapy practice office. The physical therapist was trained in neurodevelopmental treatment. The therapist had more than 10 years' experience in pediatric physical therapy. Therapy involved a combination of physical handling techniques on mobile and stationary equipment as well as the therapist's lap with toys and play activities. Motivating Gus to initiate movement and purposeful motor actions was integrated into the NDT handling. The father participated in each therapy session and learned handling techniques, activities, and positions that reinforced the physical therapy program.

Goals and Techniques

The goals and techniques employed in the therapy program are described below.

Goal 1: Improve postural stability and control in anti-gravity postures.

Techniques:

a. In wheelbarrow position with hands on bench, elicit coactivation of trunk by providing intermittent support to abdominals and pelvis.

b. Facilitate mid-range control during transitions by slowing movement down and providing intermittent handling to trunk to stimulate tone (figure A.14).

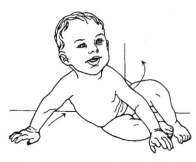

Figure A.14. Facilitate child's mid-range control during transitions by slowing down the movement and providing intermittent handling to trunk to stimulate tone.

c. Stimulate anti-gravity flexion by lowering from sit to supine and back up to sitting using trunk rotation.

Goal 2: Facilitate transitional movements and mobility skills.

Techniques:

a. Encourage lateral weight shifts while transitioning from sitting to side-sitting, to hands-and-knees position.

b. In high kneeling at bench, weight shift to side, with transitions up and down from side-sitting (figure A.15).

c. Facilitate sit to stand with forward weight shift while holding at pelvis.

d. Encourage active rolling and prone pivoting using pelvis and abdominals as key points as needed (figure A.16).

Goal 3: Stimulate use of the left body side in weight bearing patterns, trunk rotation, and use of the left arm in reaching patterns.

Techniques:

a. Encourage reaching for objects across midline by combining with weight shifts.

b. Obtain disassociation of shoulder and pelvis in prone to sit transition by providing intermittent support at scapulo-humeral region and lateral side of pelvis (figure A.17).

c. While sitting on therapist's lap, encourage child to reach behind body to get object through weight shift; apply graded pressure to abdominals and low back extensors.

Goal 4: Improve righting and equilibrium reactions in sitting.

Techniques:

a. With child sitting on therapy ball, narrow base of support of lower extremities while eliciting equilibrium reactions.

b. Stimulate righting reactions in prone, supine, and lateral head and trunk displacements during transitional movements.

Goal 5: Develop midline skills of hands.

Techniques:

a. Stimulate hand use in midline through selection of materials that encourage both hands in midline (i.e., Velcro® brand hook and loop fastener blocks, pull-apart cups).

b. Facilitate midline skills during anti-gravity flexion and sitting activities.

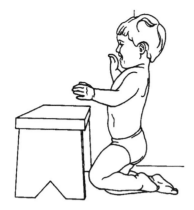

Figure A.15. The child shifts weight while high-kneeling at bench.

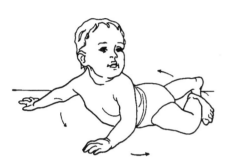

Figure A.16. Using the pelvis and abdominals, this child pivots from the prone position.

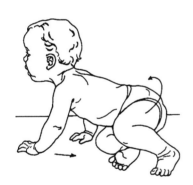

Figure A.17. The child can make a transition from prone to sit positions by obtaining intermittent support at the scapulo-humeral region and the lateral side of the pelvis.

Improvements in Skills from Pre- and Post-Assessments

1. Optical righting reactions

   Pre-assessment: Sluggish responses in prone, lateral, and supine position displacements.

   Post-assessment: Brisk responses in prone, lateral, and supine position displacement.

2. Sitting equilibriums

   Pre-assessment: Equilibriums present in lateral and anterior displacements in sitting but lacking trunk rotation component; absent in posterior direction.

   Post-assessment: Equilibriums fully developed in sitting in lateral and anterior displacements, partial neck and trunk responses in posterior direction.

3. Protective reactions in sitting

   Pre-assessment: Absence of posterior responses.

   Post-assessment: Elbow and shoulder extension components present, fingers fisted.

4. Pull to sit

   Pre-assessment: Initial head lag.

   Post-assessment: Head initiates pull to sit.

5. Tonus in trunk and extremities

   Pre-assessment: Generalized low tonus with postural fixations in symmetrical postures.

   Post-assessment: Tonus remains low throughout, but child able to hold both symmetrical and asymmetrical postures and work against gravity in low-to-ground positions.

6. Functional motor skills

   Pre-assessment: Sits when placed using wide base of support but loses balance; stepping movements present.

   Post-assessment: Pushes up into quadruped and rocks; creeps forward; sits independently and rotates trunk; rolls over supine to prone; rolls to right side; reaches overhead for toy.

7. Hand skills

   Pre-assessment: Ulnar deviation of wrists with finger hyperextension; lack of midline skills.

   Post-assessment: Holds bottle, uses pincer grasp, bangs toys in midline.

8. Sensory processing and motor planning (based on *Test of Sensory Functions in Infants*)

   Pre-assessment: Hypersensitivity to prone position; difficulty smoothly tracking a moving target or lateralizing eyes, left eye esotropia; motor planning problems.

   Post-assessment: Toleration of prone position, content on back; smooth visual tracking and lateralization of eyes; continued motor planning problems but less severe.

9. Sleep

   Pre-assessment: Needs extensive time to fall asleep, wakes frequently in the night.

   Post-assessment: Falls asleep with breast feeding only, wakes occasionally once in the night, but often sleeps through the night.

Overall Gains

When Gus' progress was examined over time, it was clear that he made good progress, but there was not a steady improvement or dramatic change over time. Table A.18 shows these results.

Gains made in parent measures were more dramatic. These are shown in table A.19.

TABLE A.18
Improvements Observed by Therapist: Gus

	1st quarter	2nd quarter	3rd quarter	4th quarter
Skill completion	13	13	16	21
Unable to complete skill	20	19	17	11

TABLE A.19
Improvements Observed by Parents: Gus

	1st quarter	2nd quarter	3rd quarter	4th quarter
Skill completion	07	17	19	27
Unable to complete skill	23	15	11	05

Gains made in specific skills observed by therapist. Gus demonstrated significant improvements in three of 12 measures completed by the therapist over time. The observation of Gus' movements out of supine were discarded since the therapist did not complete observations for this measure. The number of times that Gus was able to perform a skill during or immediately after a therapy session was tallied across the 16 sessions. Data was collected for only 13 of the 16 sessions. The results are presented in table A.20.

TABLE A.20
Gains Made in Skills Observed by Therapist: Gus

Skill	Number of Times Completed
1. Reaches to left body side in sit using trunk rotation	13/13
2. Rotates trunk to left, crossing midline with right hand	13/13
3. Assumes side-sitting on left side	11/11
4. Holds side-sitting on right over one minute	1/12
5. Rolls from supine to prone	4/13
6. Rolls to right side	6/11
7. Pivots in circle	4/13
8. Pushes up to quadruped and rocks	9/13
9. Moves forward in prone position	3/12
10. Holds object in midline	1/7
11. Holds large object and raises it overhead	0/6
12. Holds weighted toy with two hands	0/5

The last three items, involving bi-manual and midline behaviors, were not a major focus of therapy. They were also only observed in five to seven of the 16 sessions.

Gains in specific skills observed by parents. Significant progress over time was noted in three of eight behaviors in the measures observed by the parents. The results are presented in table A.21.

The skills observed by the parents that showed the most improvement over the eight weeks of therapy were holding the bottle, moving out of the backlying position, and moving forward on belly.

TABLE A.21
Gains Made in Skills Observed by Parent: Gus

Skill	Number of Times Completed
1. Holds bottle	18/26
2. Content on back	18/26
3. Rolls over	3/26
4. Does not cry and fuss when left by himself	1/26
5. Moves forward on belly	22/26
6. Holds dry cereal (oat circle) with pincer	12/26
7. Falls asleep without help	6/26
8. Wakes in the night	20/26

Description of Progress Obtained in Parent Interview

Gus' father was interviewed to determine his perception of gains in the eight-week therapy program in those areas not tapped by the daily observation measures.

Daily activities. Self-feeding is better, with independence in feeding finger foods in a reclining position. Falling and staying asleep is better. Gus is also helping out by moving body parts with dressing.

Mobility skills. Gus lifts himself up more when held and carried, and is creeping to explore his environment.

Sensory. Gus shows pleasure in moving and likes touching different textures now.

Cognitive and language. There is more interest in playing with a variety of toys, and Gus is making more vowel sounds.

Summary

Gus is a 13-month-old child with hypotonia and delayed motor development who received physical therapy twice a week for eight weeks. His presenting problems included poor postural stability and control, a tendency for postural fixations that interfered with trunk rotation and transitional movements, difficulty using the left body side, poor midline skills, fine motor problems, and motor planning difficulties. Gus demonstrated significant progress in the areas of trunk rotation, use of the left body side, creeping, refined pincer grasp, and midline skills. Improvements were also noted in self-feeding and sleep, there was less hypersensitivity to the back-lying position, and better motor planning skills. This case is an example of a young child who benefitted from a short-term NDT intervention program.

Case Description 4: Jed

Jed is a 6-year-old Caucasian child with right hemiparesis. He began receiving physical therapy at 19 months, when difficulties in using his right body side were discovered. Referral was made for occupational therapy when Jed was 3½ years old, when problems with self-care, fine motor, and perceptual-motor skills became apparent. Jed continued to receive therapy until his fifth year, and since then he has been monitored rather than receiving direct treatment. His therapists, in conjunction with his parents, felt that Jed had plateaued in his motor skills. Because Jed was entering the first grade, his parents were concerned that he would have difficulty with classroom activities such as handwriting. The parents were also concerned about Jed's ability to engage in dressing skills involving fasteners and to play with his peers in playground activities. Because the parents' concerns were in areas more often addressed in occupational therapy, Jed was referred for neurodevelopmental treatment as provided by O.T. in the research project. Of particular interest was to determine whether a child who had reached a plateau in his motor skills would benefit from short-term intervention.

Pertinent History

Jed was born prematurely at 34 weeks gestation, with a birth weight of 4 lbs., 12 oz. He was shunted for hydrocephaly at 10 days. Diagnosis of right hemiparesis was made at 19 months, when a referral was made for physical therapy.

Developmental History

Jed is a bright, sociable boy who experiences difficulties in motor control of the right body side and in visual-motor perceptual skills. His gross and fine motor skills are delayed at approximately the 3½- to 4-year level.

Primary Presenting Problems (Pre-Test Observations)

The primary problems that were identified during the initial assessment are presented in table A.22.

TABLE A.22
Primary Presenting Problems: Jed

1. Asymmetrical alignment of the trunk during table top activities, involving: bilateral hand use with scapular retraction, humeral internal rotation, and lateral flexion of the trunk on the right side when sitting.

2. Difficulty stabilizing objects with the right hand while the left hand is engaged in tool use or skilled bi-manual tasks (e.g., buttoning, drawing). Movement components that are compromised in the right hand include wrist and forearm rotation, active wrist and finger extension, and ulnar deviation.

3. Difficulty with visual-motor skills in the areas of design copying, block construction, and representational drawing.

4. Poor bilateral symmetrical upper extremity use in tasks such as catching and throwing a large ball, particularly in speed and accuracy of arm and hand movements, and in sustaining the right arm in an appropriate posture of readiness to move or hold the object.

5. Sluggish equilibrium reactions in sitting and standing, with poor dynamic and static balance in tasks such as hopping, jumping, standing on one foot, or balance beam activities.

6. Weak thoracic extension during upward reach activities, and weak postural stability of the trunk.

7. Low motivation and lack of participatory interest in outdoor playground games or table top activities involving bilateral assistive hand use or visual-motor skills.

Parents' Concerns

The parents expressed concerns in the following areas:
1. Improving Jed's capacity to manipulate fasteners for independent dressing

2. Developing more competence in fine motor and visual-motor skills to allow him to keep up with his peers in classroom activities

3. Enhancing Jed's balance and agility in outdoor games (such as kicking a ball in soccer games)

4. Improving Jed's persistence and motivation in fine motor and perceptual tasks

Measures Completed by Therapist

After each therapy session, the therapist observed the behaviors listed in table A.23.

TABLE A.23
Measures Completed by Therapist: Jed

1.	Sits with symmetrical trunk alignment during table top tasks involving two hands while seated on a therapy bench or similar furniture up to two minutes:	Y N
2.	Holds paper steadily with right hand while drawing with his left up to 30 seconds:	Y N
3.	Cuts a corner or angle (triangle or square edge) with the scissors (indicating ability to reposition paper with right hand):	Y N
4.	Holds a stencil with right hand while tracing shape with left:	Y N
5.	Buttons small buttons:	Y N
6.	Shoe tying	
	—Ties first knot:	Y N
	—Forms bunny ear loops:	Y N
	—Crosses bunny ear loops:	Y N
	—Ties bunny ear loops in knot:	Y N
7.	Visual-motor	
	—Initiates draw-a-person on his own:	Y N
	—Copies diagonal lines (X or triangle):	Y N
8.	Sits at table for visual-motor, visual perceptual, and fine motor activities (indicating attention span) for how long in session before wanting to leave table: _____	
9.	Standing balance	
	—Stands on right foot alone for how long? _____	
	—Stands on left foot alone for how long? _____	
10.	Hops on left foot how many times? _____	
11.	Catches ball with both hands and body:	Y N

Log Completed by Parents

Jed's parents entered their observations in a log two or three times a week during the course of therapy. The behaviors they looked for are presented in table A.24 (see page 98).

Description of the Therapy Program

Jed was treated twice a week in one-hour sessions over the course of eight weeks by an occupational therapist trained in neurodevelopmental treatment. The therapist had more than 10 years' experience working with children with motor impairments and in the application of neurodevelopmental treatment. Therapy was provided in a center-based, outpatient therapy setting. The emphasis in therapy was on direct physical handling, facilitation of movement patterns and skills through verbal monitoring and specific positions and activities, and home programming. The therapist used a variety of handling techniques, including mobile equipment, positioning for seating on therapy benches, and upper extremity and hand handling. Key points used were primary trunk, pelvis, shoulders, forearm, and wrist. Toys and activities were used to motivate Jed to engage in functional self-care and bilateral assistive tasks.

TABLE A.24
Log Completed by Parents: Jed

1. Buttons buttons:	Y N
—On clothing on self?	Y N
—On doll or other person?	Y N
Size: Small ($^{1}/_{2}$") _____ Medium ($^{3}/_{4}$") _____	
2. Ties shoes:	Y N
—Ties first knot:	Y N
—Forms bunny ear loops:	Y N
—Crosses bunny ear loops:	Y N
—Ties bunny ear loops in knot:	Y N
3. Zips zipper on jacket:	Y N
—Aligns zipper into placket:	Y N
—Pulls zipper up all the way to top using left hand:	Y N
—Needs reminder to hold with right hand:	Y N
4. Sits with symmetrical trunk alignment during table top tasks involving two hands while seated on a therapy bench up to two minutes:	Y N
5. Sits at table for visual-motor, visual perceptual, and fine motor activities for how long before wanting to leave table? _____	
6. Catches ball with both hands and body:	Y N
7. Plays outdoor games such as kicking ball in soccer game, throwing ball into basket, running games of tag, or hitting a ball with baseball bat	
—For how long? _____	
—What games did he like? _____	

Goals and Techniques

Goal 1: Improve symmetrical alignment of the trunk during bilateral upper extremity activities.

Techniques:

    a. Positioning on therapy bench in sitting; obtaining symmetry of trunk through the use of incline, table, and wall surfaces during two-handed activities such as kneading clay dough or using a rolling pin.

    b. Visual monitoring through use of mirror and verbal cuing, along with intermittent readjustments of trunk manually by therapist to obtain trunk symmetry.

Goal 2: Improve use of the right hand as an efficient stabilizer during bilateral assistive tasks.

Techniques:

    a. Throw balls overhead using two hands to activate forearm, wrist, and hand alignment in combination with trunk extension.

    b. Improve range in right hand, using weight bearing to obtain wrist extension, and palmar spreading to obtain palmar extension.

    c. While prone on ball, cut styrofoam blocks in half using a dull saw.

    d. Standing at chalkboard, wipe blackboard clear (with both hands using cloth or big sponge).

Goal 3: Improve visual-motor skills.

Techniques:

    a. Build block constructions in large-movement activities (i.e., pick up objects placed in different body orientations, then put into configuration).

    b. Engage in chalkboard drawing activities that use both left and right hands (i.e., simultaneous circles).

    c. Create visual patterns using streamers held with both hands (i.e., diagonals, vertical lines, zigzags).

Goal 4: Improve dynamic and static standing balance.

Techniques:

    a. Focus on weight-bearing and weight shifting to right while sitting on therapy ball.

    b. In standing, throw balls to various targets in room while weight shifting to right side (figure A.18).

    c. Using facilitation at the calf and ankle, obtain supported standing on right foot while left foot is engaged in kicking ball or lifting in air (figure A.19).

    d. Walk along uneven surfaces (e.g., pillows, air mattress) while picking up objects on floor with which to build.

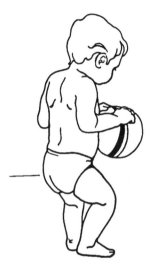

Figure A.18. Throwing a ball from a standing position helps the child improve both dynamic and standing balance.

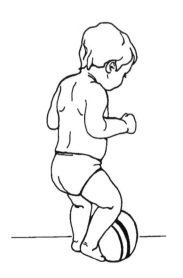

Figure A.19. While one foot kicks the ball, the other supports the child's weight through facilitation at the calf and ankle.

Improvements in Skills from Pre- to Post-Assessments

1. Trunk posture during table-top activities

    Pre-assessment: Asymmetrical, with trunk leaning to right when sitting on therapy bench and engaged in bilateral upper extremity tasks.

    Post-assessment: Maintenance of symmetrical trunk posture 85% of the time when sitting on therapy bench.

2. Use of right hand as an efficient stabilizer during bilateral assistive tasks

    Pre-assessment: Static use of the right hand in holding objects that require readjustment (e.g., holding string for stringing beads) with hyper-extension at the metacarpals and ulnar deviation of wrist; inability to hold objects steadily with right hand (e.g., cannot hold paper while drawing with left hand).

    Post-assessment: Readjusts objects in right hand, showing improved in-hand manipulation and stabilization of metacarpals—resulting in improvements in skill performance (e.g., buttoning); ability to hold paper down with loosely fisted right hand.

3. Development of bilateral skills

    Pre-assessment: Can unbutton large buttons, unscrew jar lid, and cut 6" line; unable to button large button, cut 2" triangle with 1/2" accuracy, catch 9" ball with arms and body, zip a zipper or string beads with efficient speed and accuracy (e.g., strings four 1/2" beads in two minutes), or tie shoelaces.

    Post-assessment: Able to string beads, cut 2" triangle with 1/2" accuracy; catch 9" ball with hands and body; zip a zipper; string seven 1/2" beads in two minutes. Ties first knot in shoe tying.

4. Develop visual-motor skills

    Pre-assessment: Able to imitate a cross but cannot copy a cross from a model; and unable to draw a man or other representational figure.

    Post-assessment: Copies a cross; draws a representation of a man with head, body, arms, legs, and some facial features; shows interest in drawing and spontaneously initiates drawing.

5. Develop standing balance

    Pre-assessment: Stands on right foot momentarily and on left foot for only three seconds; has difficulty walking on a balance beam; is unable to hop on left foot.

    Post-assessment: Stands on left foot for 10 seconds and on right foot for one second; walks on an 8-foot balance beam without stepping off; hops on left foot two times.

Overall Gains

Significant progress was found overall in skills observed by the therapist as well as the parents. The 16 therapy sessions were divided into four equal periods and the data were inspected for presence or absence of skill completion. This procedure was used for the parent observations also. The therapist-generated results are displayed in table A.25.

Measures collected by the parents also showed gains. Table A.26 presents those results.

TABLE A.25
Improvements Observed by Therapist: Jed

	1st quarter	2nd quarter	3rd quarter	4th quarter
Skill completion	12	23	23	27
Unable to complete skill	36	25	25	21

TABLE A.26
Improvements Observed by Parents: Jed

	1st quarter	2nd quarter	3rd quarter	4th quarter
Skill completion	3	12	28	36
Unable to complete skill	39	30	7	6

Gains made in specific skills observed by therapist. The number of times that Jed was able to perform a skill during or immediately after a therapy session were tallied across the 16 sessions. Because Jed had not had therapy in more than a year and he was an older child, it was not expected that he would show quick and immediate results in skill performance. However, when comparisons were made between pre- and post-test performance, all of the skills were absent on pre-test and present on post-test. Table A.27 (see page 102) presents the findings for frequency and change from pre- to post-test.

Gains made in specific skills observed by parents. Changes were found in all skills observed by the parents. The observation of "sitting with symmetrical trunk" was discarded because the parents did not observe it. The results are displayed in table A.28 (see page 102).

TABLE A.27
Gains Made in Skills Observed by Therapist: Jed

Skill	Number of Times Completed
1. Sits with symmetrical trunk	11/16
2. Holds paper steadily	8/16
3. Cuts angles with scissors	8/16
4. Holds stencil with right hand	3/16
5. Buttons medium buttons	4/16
6. Ties first knot in shoe tying	6/16
7. Draws a person	4/16
8. Copies cross or triangle	4/16
9. Sits for > 10 minutes at table top tasks	12/16
10. Catches ball with hands and body	6/16

TABLE A.28
Gains Made in Skills Observed by Parents: Jed

Skill	Number of Times Completed
1. Buttons medium buttons	18/23
2. Ties first knot in shoe tying	14/23
3. Pulls zipper to top on jacket	13/23
4. Sits at table for more than 10 minutes	12/23
5. Catches ball with hands and body	13/23
6. Plays outdoor games for over 10 minutes	8/23

Description of Progress Obtained in Parent Interview

Jed's mother was interviewed to determine the ways she felt that Jed had improved during the eight-week therapy program in areas not captured by the daily observations. She said that Jed had developed a new interest in playing outdoors as his balance and bilateral coordination improved. He could pump his bicycle pedals, propelling the bicycle (with training wheels) up hills. He was interested in riding a swing and could hold on to the swing ropes with both hands, but could not yet pump his feet to make the swing go. Overall, Jed was showing much more confidence in his skills, playing longer at the table during perceptual and fine motor tasks, and doing much more for himself in self-care.

Summary

At the conclusion of the therapy program, Jed had demonstrated significant progress in bilateral upper extremity development, dynamic and static balance, hand use, self-care, and visual–motor skills. Substantial gains were found in all skills tested between the pre- and post-test. Jed developed more confidence in his abilities and began to initiate outdoor games and table top activities (e.g., perceptual and fine motor) spontaneously. These were activities that he had avoided prior to the therapy program. This case points to the importance of providing short-term therapy to older children even after they seem to have plateaued in their skills. Doing so can help determine whether additional therapy intervention might be helpful.

Case Description 5: Alicia

Alicia is a 2-year-old child of Hispanic descent with spastic diplegia. She has received specialized therapy services through the county school system's early intervention program since she was eight months old. In addition, Alicia has received ongoing physical therapy once a week. Because Alicia's primary motor problems are in gross motor skills and the parents are most concerned about her learning to walk, physical therapy was provided as part of the research project. Alicia did not have orthotics at the onset of the therapy. By the end of therapy, she had been fitted with supra-malleolar orthotics. She had not worn them consistently or long enough for her therapist to consider them a variable that affected performance, however.

Pertinent History

Alicia was born at 28 weeks gestation because of a premature rupture of membranes. She weighed 3 lbs. at birth. Alicia experienced multiple neonatal complications, including respiratory distress syndrome.

Developmental History

Alicia is a very bright little girl who functions at age level in her cognitive, social-emotional, language, and fine motor skills, which was confirmed by developmental testing. Her gross motor skills fall at approximately the 10-month level.

Primary Presenting Problems
(Pre-Test Observations)

Alicia's primary problems, identified during the pre–test, are presented in table A.29.

TABLE A.29
Primary Presenting Problems: Alicia

1. Lack of graded flexion/extension of the lower extremities in standing; inability to lower self slowly to squatting.

2. Inadequate trunk and pelvic rotation in transitional movements with difficulty tolerating side-sitting position to either side, in utilizing rotation to get in and out of a chair, or to reach behind back for a toy; static weight shifts of pelvis.

3. Limited thoracic extension in upward reach while sitting in a chair; scapulo-humeral tightness with mild scapular protraction and humeral internal rotation; thoracic rounding in sitting.

4. Predominance of flexor posture of upper extremities in assisted walking.

5. Pattern of plantar flexion, inversion, and pronation of feet in standing and in assisted walking; lack of heel strike; more toeing-in of right foot.

6. Poor static and dynamic balance in standing, with inability to stand alone; strong fear response to falling.

7. Delayed equilibrium reactions in sitting, with sluggish responses and incomplete trunk rotation.

8. Strong posterior tilt pattern of pelvis in long sitting with shortening of the hamstrings; preference for W-sitting pattern.

9. Weak proximal stability of the trunk, specifically weak abdominals and mid- and low-back extensors; strong lordotic posture of trunk in kneeling and standing positions.

10. Poor disassociation of the lower extremities, particularly when the right leg initiates movement; able to move from half-kneel to stand on left but not right leg; creeps with some disassociation of legs; incomplete hip extension in kneeling and standing.

11. Increased tonus in pelvis and lower extremities with significant underlying weakness in the trunk and lower extremities; strong tendency to over-use upper extremities.

12. Decreased desire to move and explore the environment.

Parents' Concerns

Her parents were most concerned that Alicia learn to stand and walk. They are very motivated to help their daughter and have been intimately involved in her therapy program.

Measures Completed by the Therapist

The measures completed by the therapist were documented after each therapy session. Table A.30 presents the measures.

TABLE A.30
Measures Completed by Therapist: Alicia

1. Develop graded flexion/extension of lower extremities in standing.
   a. Lowers self slowly to squat position to pick up toys on floor: Y N
   b. Holds bear position while reaching for toys between legs and out to body sides: Y N
      Requires:
      Minimal assist _____
      Maximal assist _____
      No assist _____

2. Improve trunk rotation in various developmental positions.
   a. Gets in and out of child-sized chair using trunk rotation: Y N
   b. Holds side-sitting position while reaching up and across body diagonally: Y N

3. Improve thoracic extension in developmental positions.
   a. While sitting on bench with feet supported, Alicia reaches upward with both hands to grasp large object; thoracic spine is extended: Y N
   b. Alicia reaches behind herself to obtain toy while long sitting using trunk rotation: Y N

4. Decrease flexion pattern in upper extremities during assisted walking.
   a. Arms can be extended fully overhead during assisted walking (no elbow flexion or pulling into flexion of arms felt): Y N
   b. Alicia can hold a large foam ball with two hands in relaxed upper extremity position while gait is facilitated at pelvis: Y N

5. Inhibit plantarflexion and inversion pattern of feet during assisted walking.
   a. While walking a distance of 15 feet, feet remain parallel, with heels down.
      —with orthotics: Y N
      —without orthotics: Y N

6. Improve balance.
   a. Stands momentarily by herself: Y N
   b. Stands momentarily without fear response: Y N
   c. Equilibrium reactions in sitting show complete trunk rotation to both sides: Y N
   d. Balance reactions are brisk and automatic in sitting: Y N

Log Completed By Parents

The parents entered their own observations in a log two or three times a week during the course of the therapy program. The behaviors they looked for are presented in table A.31 (see page 108).

TABLE A.31
Log Completed by Parents: Alicia

1.	When standing at table, will pick up toy on floor, then go back up to stand:	Y	N

2. Ask Alicia to "sit correctly," then watch her to see if she stays in this position (*without* encouraging her).

a.	Sits cross legged:	Y	N
b.	Long sits:	Y	N
c.	Side sits:	Y	N
d.	W-sits:	Y	N

3. If placed in side-sitting position, how long will she play this way without needing help? (Maximum five minutes each side; it may only be a very short time each side.)
   a. On right side: _____
   b. On left side: _____

4.	When walking her with arms stretched out overhead across room, arms feel relaxed and do not pull into flexion:	Y	N

5.	Stands alone:	Y	N

   a. How long? _____

b.	She was without fear when you let go of her:	Y	N
6.	Walks with heels down and with feet pointing straight out during assisted walking across room:	Y	N

Description of the Therapy Program

Alicia was treated twice a week in one-hour sessions over the course of eight weeks by a physical therapist trained in neurodevelopmental treatment. The therapist had more than 10 years' experience in working with children with motor impairments, and in the application of neurodevelopmental treatment. All therapy sessions were provided in the home. The emphasis in therapy was on direct physical handling and home programming. The therapist employed a variety of handling techniques, including the use of mobile equipment, therapy benches, and toys. Key points of control were primarily trunk and pelvis. The therapist provided direct proprioceptive input to the feet. In addition, upper extremity posture was facilitated through positioning of the task (i.e., reaching upward for a toy; carrying a 9" ball). Toys and activities were used to motivate proper body alignment, reach patterns, and lower extremity movements.

Goals and Techniques

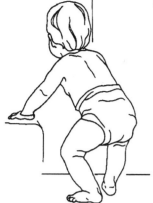

Figure A.20. Moving slowly from squat to stand and back again helps the child improve flexion and extension of the lower extremities.

Goal 1: Improve graded flexion/extension of the lower extremities.

Techniques:

a. While standing with proper trunk and lower extremity alignment, facilitate movement to squat or reaching to floor, then back to stand. Guide pelvis initially; there is a decreasing need for pelvic control over time if movement is completed slowly and with control (figure A.20).

b. Facilitate squat to stand with feet in parallel and symmetrical alignment, as well as with one foot in front of the other. This improves control in movement, while putting differing demands on pelvis and lower extremities.

c. Using a bear position with hands on varying surfaces (e.g., therapy benches of differing heights), help child practice reaching between legs for toy on floor. Vary placement of toy to obtain weight shifts in feet and pelvic rotation, then put toy on bench, all the time controlling at pelvis and on quadriceps as key points (figure A.21).

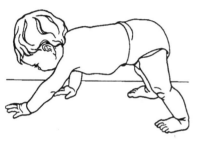

Figure A.21. The child demonstrates the bear position on an even surface.

Goal 2: Improve trunk and pelvic rotation in transitional movements.

Techniques:

a. Prepare trunk and pelvis for rotation by placing child prone on therapy ball, arms extended overhead and pelvis extended, with hips abducted; weight shift laterally then as pelvis begins to free in its range. Disassociating pelvis from trunk, rotate child's pelvis to sidelying position and elicit active trunk movements to laterally flex and sit up to semi side-sitting.

b. On therapy ball or on floor, stimulate child's transitions, including supine to side-lying to side-sit; prone to quadruped to side-sit, and supine to long sit to side-sit, always monitoring or controlling pelvis to obtain pelvic rotation and trunk-pelvis disassociation.

c. In long sitting or sitting on therapy bench, encourage child to reach behind the body for toys to obtain upper and mid-trunk rotation. Sustain pelvis in proper tilt (e.g., not posterior tilt) and maintain lower extremities in posture so that hamstrings are lengthened and/or feet are dorsiflexed.

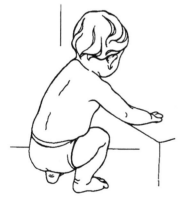

Figure A.22. This child lowers self from standing to sit, relying on furniture for support.

d. Have child practice lowering self from standing to sit in a chair or on a bench (figure A.22). Movement should proceed in a slow, graded fashion while rotating the pelvis. Arms may be overhead on therapist's shoulders.

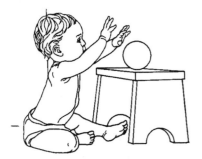

Figure A.23. The child demonstrates thoracic extension while reaching for objects.

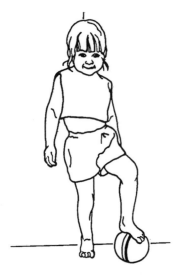

Figure A.24. The child demonstrates weight bearing with one foot on the ball while the other foot supports standing.

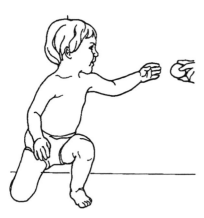

Figure A.25. Reaching for the ball, the child demonstrates weight shifting from a half-kneel position.

Goal 3: Improve thoracic extension while lengthening the scapulo-humeral region and inhibiting flexor pattern of upper extremities.

Techniques:

a. Obtain thoracic extension and upward reach by using wall surfaces, high benches, or a large therapy ball for reaching (figure A.23). Maintain control when necessary on abdominals and low back extensors, or provide cues for elbow extension and upward reach at triceps or at scapula when necessary. Work in various developmental positions.

b. While child is prone on therapy ball, activate thoracic and elbow extensors through weight bearing on hands. Hold child at pelvis and weight shift forward-back and laterally, then stimulate stepping on hands, or reaching with one hand while the other bears weight.

c. In standing and walking, engage Alicia in holding large objects (e.g., 9" ball) to inhibit flexor posture, or in tasks involving bilateral upward reach (e.g., lifting hand overhead).

Goal 4: Obtain complete range of motion in the hip flexors, hamstrings, and ankle dorsiflexors, then activate hip extensors and ankle dorsiflexion with leg disassociation.

Techniques:

a. Gently range child's hips and ankles, providing sustained stretch with deep proprioceptive input through heels into quadriceps, gastric, and gluteals. While maintaining range, follow with weight bearing into lower extremity to activate pattern.

b. Use weight shifts and weight bearing in positions, including: one foot up on stool or small ball while standing; kneel to half-kneel to stand; standing with one foot in front of other (figures A.24 and A.25). Take care to inhibit knee recurvatem.

Goal 5: Improve equilibrium reactions, with emphasis on active trunk and pelvis rotations.

Techniques:

a. While holding child at pelvis in sit position on therapy ball, elicit equilibrium reactions in various planes with different speeds, always monitoring pelvis to avoid posterior tilt.

b. Stimulate equilibriums in standing by putting one foot in therapist's hand while other remains on floor. Holding child's foot, move in various planes to activate responses in fore-foot.

Goal 6: Develop proximal stability of the trunk.

Techniques:

 a. Using transitional movements (e.g., supine to sit), facilitate holding of abdominal and back extensors by using techniques such as sweep tapping on the abdominals, or holding in mid-positions.

 b. Focus on anti-gravity postures of flexion and extension in positions and activities previously described.

Goal 7: Facilitate gait patterns in assisted walking.

Techniques:

 a. Controlling at the pelvis, encourage child to take slow steps with heel down and foot in parallel alignment in moving forward, side, and backwards.

 b. Facilitate gait at pelvis while child holds small ball to inhibit arm flexion.

Improvements in Skills from Pre- to Post-Assessments

1. Lower extremity skills

   Pre-assessment: Stands at furniture on toes or with knees locked; unable to reach to floor for toy or to squat in play; cruises one to two steps using high steppage pattern; pulls to stand through half kneeling; creeping is primary mode of movement; unable to stand alone.

   Post-assessment: Stands at furniture with heels in contact with floor and without knee recurvatem; knee walks; cruises freely at wall or at furniture; walks pushing a cart or a pull walker; right foot continues to turn inward, with most of weight on left; stance is more erect with hip extension; stands alone from five to 10 seconds.

2. Sitting posture

   Pre-assessment: Sits in long sit with posterior pelvic tilt, thoracic rounding, and elevated shoulders; strong preference for W-sitting; unable to side-sit; very symmetrical trunk.

   Post-assessment: Continues to long sit with posterior pelvic tilt and thoracic rounding; side-sits spontaneously on occasion and holds position briefly in play or uses as a transition; automatically sits in either long sit or side-sit; uses trunk rotation in transitions and assumes asymmetrical body postures rather than always staying very symmetrical.

3. Equilibrium reactions

   Pre-assessment: Sluggish in sitting, with only partial trunk rotation; no equilibriums in standing.

   Post-assessment: Brisk and automatic in sitting, with complete trunk rotation; foot responses emergent in standing balance.

4. Upper extremity posture in standing

   Pre-assessment: Arms flexed at elbows, with humeral internal rotation and shoulder protraction in standing; scapulo-humeral tightness with limited overhead reach (120°).

   Post-assessment: Arms free to reach in various planes while standing; elbows occasionally flexed; able to reach overhead to full range while standing.

5. Lower extremity alignment

   Pre-assessment: Tightness in hip flexors, hamstrings, and plantar flexors; foot pronation and inversion, with more toeing-in on right; strong posterior tilt of pelvis; unable to put heel completely down in standing.

   Post-assessment: Complete range attained in hip flexors; hamstrings remain tight; heel can bear weight in stand with improved range (gain of 15-20°); right foot continues to toe in; posterior tilt of pelvis present, but now can weight shift over pelvis and rotate pelvis in transitional movements.

Overall Gains

Significant progress overall was found in skills that were documented by the therapist and by the parents. The 16 therapy sessions were divided into groups of four sessions each and the data were inspected for improvements over time. The parent observations were divided into quarters and analyzed similarly. Tables A.32 and A.33 document the results.

TABLE A.32
Improvements Observed by Therapist: Alicia

	1st quarter	2nd quarter	3rd quarter	4th quarter
Skill completion	23	37	40	51
Unable to complete skill	29	15	12	1

TABLE A.33
Improvements Observed by Parents: Alicia

	1st quarter	2nd quarter	3rd quarter	4th quarter
Skill completion	19	24	30	31
Unable to complete skill	11	11	4	1

Gains made in specific skills observed by therapist. Alicia demonstrated gains in eight of the 13 measures. An additional two skills—reaching behind the back in long sitting, and standing momentarily without fear—had improved significantly when progress was examined over time. The results are presented in table A.34.

TABLE A.34
Gains Made in Skills Observed by Therapist: Alicia

Skill	Number of Times Completed
1. Lowers self to squat to pick up toy	13/16
2. Holds bear position without help	3/16
3. Rotates trunk to get in and out of chair	16/16
4. Holds side-sit	14/16
5. Reaches up overhead with thoracic extension	16/16
6. Reaches behind trunk while long sitting	11/16
7. Walks with arms extended overhead in assisted walking (no elbow flexion)	9/16
8. Holds ball with two hands while assisted in walking	9/16
9. Walks with feet parallel and heels down in assisted gait	12/16
10. Stands momentarily	12/16
11. Stands momentarily without fear response	6/16
12. Rotates trunk in sitting equilibrium	13/16
13. Equilibrium responses are brisk and automatic in sitting	14/16

Gains made in specific skills observed by parents. Significant changes in specific skills were observed by the parents in four of the seven measures. Two additional measures showed progress over time. The observations of side-sitting were not recorded by the parents and discarded from the analysis. Sitting posture was captured in the "sits correctly" measure. In addition, the parents broke apart observations of walking with feet straight and walking with heels down, making this two measures instead of one. Table A.35 (see page 114) presents these findings.

The "sits correctly" measure consisted of long sitting as a preferred posture, although side sitting was observed a few times. Interestingly, improvements were found for arm posture (lack of elbow flexion) in walking with arms overhead by the parents, but not by the therapist. It is possible that the parents were less observant of elbow flexion when present, or that more elbow flexion occurred with the therapist because her facilitation of gait was more demanding.

TABLE A.35
Gains Made in Skills Observed by Parents: Alicia

Skill	Number of Times Completed
1. Picks up toy from floor when standing	14/14
2. Sits "correctly" (no W-sitting)	11/14
3. Walks with arms overhead without elbow flexion	12/14
4. Stands alone for at least three seconds	7/14
5. Shows no fear of falling in standing	3/14
6. Walks with heels down	14/14
7. Walks with feet straight	10/14

Two skills showed improvement over time: "stands alone over three seconds," and "walks with feet straight."

Description of Progress Obtained in Parent Interview

Alicia's mother was interviewed following the eight-week therapy program to determine if any progress was made in areas not directly measured in the assessments. She stated that Alicia had a strong desire to walk where previously she was content to creep about. She walks with a more erect body and her hands down.

Since her balance has improved, Alicia is comfortable standing next to other children who may bump or jostle her in play. On her own, Alicia will sit "right"—"they don't have to fight about it"; there are "no complaints." Alicia reaches more with both hands; before, she preferred to use only her left hand. In addition, Alicia helps more with dressing herself and has gained more control in using the spoon.

Summary

Alicia is a 2-year-old girl with spastic diplegia who demonstrated significant progress toward independent standing and walking in the 8-week physical therapy NDT program. Major changes were observed in the areas of lower extremity, function, standing balance, equilibrium reactions in sitting, foot alignment in standing and assisted gait, trunk and pelvic rotation; arm posture in standing and walking, and sitting posture. Significant progress was documented both in overall progress over the eight-week program and in attainment of specific skills.

Case Description 6: Willa

Willa is a 2-year-old child of black-Caucasian descent with a diagnosis of spastic quadriplegia. She currently attends a school-based program that provides individualized therapy services in addition to the educational program. Willa began occupational therapy services at 10 months of age and entered the school-based program at 13 months.

Pertinent History

Willa was born prematurely, at 28 weeks, with a birth weight of 2 lbs., 3 oz. She received ventilation for six weeks. She developed hydrocephalus due to an intraventricular hemorrhage for which she was shunted. Because of repeated shunt infections, Willa has had eight shunt revisions. Willa also had retinopathy of prematurity and has mild esotropia of the right eye.

Developmental History

Overall, Willa is functioning at the 3- to 4-month level in motor and cognitive skills. Language skill assessment placed Willa at the 5-month level. Her strength is in social emotional skills, which range from the 3- to 7-month level. In the past year at her school-based program, Willa has shown little change in her developmental status.

Primary Presenting Problems (Pre-Test Observations)

The primary problems identified during the assessment are presented on table A.36 (see page 116).

Other problems that were noted were difficulties with oral motor control (e.g., poor lip closure on spoon, drooling, immature chewing pattern with suckling pattern); and limited sound production with capacity to produce vowel sounds only. Difficulties with self-calming were reported by the parents in addition to distress at being dressed and bathed. Distractibility to sounds and sights were also noted.

TABLE A.36
Primary Presenting Problems: Willa

1. Increased hypertonus in the right upper extremity, trunk, and both lower extremities with limited range in the hamstrings.

2. Limited use and awareness of the right upper extremity; tightly fisted and inactive right arm; ability to reach with left hand for easily obtainable objects but exploration (e.g., shake or inspect) is limited in left hand.

3. Predominance of the ATNR in supine and supported sitting to the right side.

4. Inability to reach for feet and tuck neck in supine, to roll from back to stomach toward left, or to weight shift while prone on elbows, particularly to right side.

5. Difficulty isolating head movements from trunk in supported sitting with reliance upon arm propping and shoulder elevation pattern.

6. Strong positive supporting reflex of legs with plantar flexion in standing and strong extensor tone in legs in supported sitting.

7. Weak neck and trunk stability with some head lag on pull to sit and poor to fair head control in supported sitting.

Parents' Concerns

The primary areas of concern identified by the parents included:
1. Sound production
2. Rolling over
3. Sitting and crawling
4. Reaching and use of right arm

Measures Completed by the Therapist

The measures completed by the therapist following each session are presented in table A.37.

TABLE A.37
Measures Completed by Therapist: Willa

1. Improve use and awareness of right hand.
   a. Reaches for foot: Y N
   b. Uses reaching movements for interesting toy (left hand may also reach):   Y N
   c. Holds both hands in midline in play: Y N
   d. Takes toy from right hand to manipulate with left: Y N

2. Inhibit ATNR in developmental positions.
   a. When backlying, reaches for feet and/or keeps head centered, arms in midline: Y N
   b. In supported sitting, engages in midline play without ATNR: Y N

3. Improve mobility skills.
   a. Rolls from back to stomach toward left side: Y N
   b. When left by herself on mat for three minutes, will roll over if encouraged: Y N
   Number of times _____

TABLE A.37 (continued)
Measures Completed by Therapist: Willa

4. Develop independent sitting without shoulder elevation pattern.
   a. When placed in circle sit, will turn head to look to either side at interesting toy: Y   N
   b. When sitting on floor with arms resting on low bench surface, will reach with left hand for toy: Y   N
      Presence of shoulder elevation: Y   N

5. Improve left-hand manipulation of toys.
   a. Shakes rattle in left hand: Y   N
   b. Turns object over in left hand to inspect (e.g., bell):   Y   N

6. Improve prone propping and weight shift in prone.
   a. Will lean onto right arm to reach for toy, with left placed across midline: Y   N
   b. Will weight shift onto left arm in prone (e.g., looks to right side): Y   N

Log Developed for Parent Observations

A set of observations were developed for use by the parents; however, because they were lost, they were not included in the progress analysis of this case. Since the behavioral observations are still useful as examples for other cases, they are presented in table A.38.

TABLE A.38
Log Completed by Parents: Willa

1. Imitates sounds in games like peek-a-boo: Y   N

2. When placed on floor, rolls over with encouragement (for interesting toy, etc.) (Three-minute observation):   Y   N
   —Number of times she rolled: _____

3. When placed in circle sitting position, arms on floor, will watch balls or cars rolling from left to right and back without falling over: Y   N

4. Plays with feet with both hands: Y   N

5. Shakes and manipulates a toy in her left hand: Y   N

6. Moves her right hand when touched with interesting texture (i.e., soft ball, rough hair brush, placed in bin of dried beans):   Y   N
   —Opens hand after sensory stimulation: Y   N

7. Holds large objects (e.g., ball) with both hands in middle of body: Y   N

8. Closes lips around spoon when fed pureed foods: Y   N
   —If given pressure at lower lip: Y   N

9. Healthy and feeling good on day of observation: Y   N

Description of the Therapy Program

Willa was treated twice a week in 30-minute sessions over the course of eight weeks by a physical therapist trained in neurodevelopmental treatment. The therapist had more than ten years' experience in working with children with motor impairments and in the application of neurodevelopmental treatment. Therapy was provided at a school in a self-contained therapy room. Consultation to the parents and classroom teacher was provided. It focused on positioning for feeding, fine motor, and learning activities. Everyday management activities were emphasized, such as proper ways to carry, dress, bathe, and feed Willa. The physical therapy sessions involved direct physical handling and included handling on the therapist's lap, on mobile equipment, and on the mat. Therapy benches were used to facilitate sitting posture and upper extremity use in upright positions. Toys and activities were used to motivate Willa to move or engage in functional tasks. Easy-to-grasp toys and visually interesting materials were used.

Goals and Techniques

Goal 1: Improve antigravity flexion to allow for reaching toward feet, midline hand use, and rolling.

Techniques:

a. In supine or on therapist's lap, facilitate hands to feet, hands to mouth, and hands to head through self-massage and simple reach activities.

b. Focus on elongation of thoracic extensors while activating trunk flexors, using graded sustained deep pressure and sweep tapping.

Goal 2: Improve mid-range control of head in supported sitting.

Technique:

Using graded sustained deep pressure applied to thoracic extensors and abdominals, activate mid-range control in supported sitting. Apply downward pressure to sternum to stimulate neck flexion as needed.

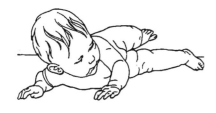

Figure A.26. This child demonstrates segmented rolling from prone to supine.

Goal 3: Improve disassociation of neck from shoulders to allow for head turning and rolling and disassociation of lower extremities, one from the other.

Techniques:

a. Stimulate shoulder depression by bringing child's hands down toward pelvis or knees in supine.

b. Stimulate sidelying to supine; sidelying to prone; and transitions up to sitting from sidelying, while keeping legs separated.

c. Stimulate segmental rolling from prone to supine (figure A.26).

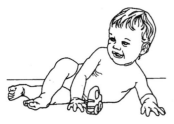

Figure A.27. This child demonstrates weight bearing on one foot while in a sidelying position.

d. Obtain weight bearing on one foot in sidelying to obtain lower extremity disassociation (figure A.27).

Goal 4: Improve sensory awareness.
Techniques:

   a. With child on therapist's lap while in supine, encourage the exploration of hands to body parts.

   b. Provide vestibular stimulation through rotary and linear movement on therapist's lap.

   c. Elicit sound play through tapping of hand on mouth and hand or foot on mat surface.

Goal 5: Improve use of hands.
Techniques:

   a. Encourage hands to midline by providing support at the scapular-humeral region.

   b. Stimulate crossing midline to reach for easy-to-grasp ball.

   c. Utilize weight bearing on hand as an inhibitory technique, followed by reaching with hand that had been weight bearing.

   d. Reach for toy in sidelying position; enhance midline play in this position as well as in supine.

Goal 6: Improve functional motor skills.
Techniques:

   a. Encourage lateral head righting and segmental movement in rolling from prone to supine.

   b. While in prone, facilitate weight shifts and propping prone on elbows through the use of pressure on the abdominals.

   c. Stimulate weight shifts in supported sitting to improve head control.

Improvements in Skills from Pre- to Post-Assessments

1. Use of upper extremities

   Pre-assessment: Right hand tightly fisted, inactive in reach or grasp. Left hand grasps toy, but with non-active manipulations.

   Post-assessment: Reaches and grasps toy with right hand, shakes toy; opens hand voluntarily; fisted only intermittently or loosely fisted; brings both hands to midline in play; left hand shakes rattle and inspects toy by turning over, using wrist rotation.

2. Predominance of ATNR

   Pre-assessment: Frequent obligatory ATNR positioning in supine and supported sitting to right.

   Post-assessment: Midline play and reaches for feet in supine; sits with capacity to turn head to either side; ATNR not observed.

3. Mobility skills

   Pre-assessment: Rolls only from back to stomach toward right; limited weight shift in prone, toward left only.

   Post-assessment: Rolls from back to stomach on both sides and initiates rolling spontaneously. Weight shifts to right side to reach with left hand in prone on elbows; pivots on stomach to obtain toy.

4. Head and trunk control

   Pre-assessment: Initial head lag on pull to sit; shoulder elevation pattern in supported sit is used to assist in holding posture; neck instability appears in upright position with neck hyperextension; sits propped on both arms momentarily while leaning to right; has difficulty maintaining head in midline while in prone position, with head hyperextended at times.

   Post-assessment: Initiates neck tuck on pull to sit: shoulders remain elevated in supported sitting but trunk is symmetrical; head is steady, with ability to look to either side in supported sitting; sits with arms propped; reaches while prone propping, demonstrating active weight shifts in prone.

Overall Gains Made in Therapy

Willa showed immediate gains during the first few weeks of treatment and maintained her gains over the eight weeks of treatment. Her performance is presented in table A.39.

TABLE A.39
Improvements Observed by Therapist: Willa

	1st quarter	2nd quarter	3rd quarter	4th quarter
Skill completion	52	54	57	55
Unable to complete skill	8	6	3	5

Gains made in specific skills observed by therapist. Willa demonstrated significant progress in 10 of the 15 skills observed. The number of times that Willa was able to perform a skill during or immediately after a therapy session was tallied across the 16 sessions. Table A.40 presents the findings.

TABLE A.40
Gains In Specific Skills: Willa

Skill	Number of Times Completed
1. Reaches for feet using right hand	16/16
2. Reaches for interesting toy with right hand	16/16
3. Holds hands in midline in play	16/16
4. Takes toy from right hand to manipulate in left	11/16
5. Reaches for feet in supine, keeping head centered	16/16
6. In supported sitting, plays in midline with no ATNR	16/16
7. Rolls back to stomach toward left	16/16
8. Rolls spontaneously	10/16
9. Turns head to either side in supported sitting	16/16
10. Reaches with left hand in supported sitting	16/16
11. No presence of shoulder elevation in supported sitting	0/16
12. Shakes rattle with left hand	11/16
13. Inspects object in left hand (wrist rotation)	10/16
14. Weight shifts to right to reach left in prone on elbows	15/16
15. Weight shifts to left in prone to look toward right	16/16

Description of Progress Obtained in Parent Interview

Willa's mother was interviewed to determine any improvements she had noted during the therapy program in areas that were not captured by the daily observation measures.

Motor. Willa's mother reported that Willa is using her right side much more with less fisting of the hand. She will attempt to hold a spoon with her left hand and hold a spouted cup with both hands. In prone on elbows, she uses both hands in play and stays on her elbows instead of collapsing toward her right. She sits better and doesn't slouch to the right. When she rolls, a startle no longer occurs. Willa seems aware of her feet now and reaches for them. She also feels looser and is easier to dress, bathe, and carry.

Language and communication. Willa is making more sounds, particularly consonants, and when she vocalizes, it is louder. She will call more to her baby sister and parents to let them know when she wants things. It is easier for her parents to understand what she wants and needs.

Appendix B

STRATEGIES FOR CASE STUDY RESEARCH

This appendix presents pertinent details for those who are interested in conducting case study research. First the research problem is defined, with directions for research. Some typical research questions that may be addressed using the methods in this manual are presented. Steps in conducting case study research are described, including data analyses.

Strategies for Case Study Research

The Research Problem

A major problem confronting therapists and teachers who provide services to children with neuromotor handicaps is determining the most appropriate therapy program to address the child's multiple needs. Is one therapy approach more effective than another, and with which children? This documentation is important to justify the need for therapy to referring physicians, administrators, and third-party reimbursement agencies.

Research studies examining motor intervention programs have yielded conflicting findings. (These programs include structured motor programs or specialized handling techniques—e.g., neurodevelopmental treatment—designed to ameliorate abnormal postures and movement patterns, and to promote functional motor skills.) Problems that have been identified with the research studies to date include the following:

- Instruments have tended to focus on child outcome measures (e.g., developmental performance) and are often not sensitive to indicators of change in motor performance (Ottenbacher et al. 1986; Palisano 1991; Parette and Hourcade 1984; Stern and Gorga 1988).

- The vast majority of early intervention studies have been based on subjective, clinical observations, with only 48% yielding statistical evidence of effectiveness (Palisano 1991; Simeonsson et al. 1982).

- Statistical significance is often low because of small sample sizes.

- Children often progress in domains that are not measured by the dependent variables (i.e., management areas rather than gains in developmental milestones).

- Subject characteristics are often not examined or considered in the research design (e.g., environment, parent and family traits, severity of child's handicap, and etiology).

Directions for Research

Studies are needed that investigate the *efficacy* of specific sensorimotor interventions (e.g., NDT) (Parette, Hendricks, and Rock 1991). Efficacy studies answer the question: Are gains or benefits obtained over time when an intervention is provided? Once efficacy of treatment has been established, research should focus on *effectiveness* of treatments. Effectiveness studies answer the question: Is one treatment approach more beneficial than another for which clinical populations?

The first step in research is to address efficacy. An efficacy study should investigate the following features:

- What is the treatment? To date, there are little to no conceptual or operational definitions that describe concisely what NDT is.
- When should treatment be initiated? There is evidence suggesting that the younger the child, the more responsive to treatment.
- When should treatment be ended? Termination of therapy may be related to attaining independence in self-care or mobility skills.
- At what frequency and duration should therapy be provided in order to obtain positive effects?
- Who should provide the therapy and how? Issues such as discipline of provider (i.e., OT, PT, ST, teacher); how therapy is delivered (i.e., direct treatment, consultation, parent involvement), and setting (i.e., home, clinic, school setting) need to be investigated.
- How do different disciplines providing NDT differ in their application (i.e., emphasis on ADL, feeding, play skills, mobility, etc.)?

The research model presented in this appendix represents a methodology for documenting progress as a result of therapy. The model has been tested in several clinical settings and was found useful in maintaining daily progress reports and in examining progress over time. The format for documenting changes is linked directly with therapy goals and family concerns, and therefore is very meaningful to therapist, client, and family.

Steps in Single Case Study Research

The following describes the required steps for measuring change as a result of intervention. The therapist should:

1. describe the child
2. identify the most appropriate measurement strategies for the child's primary problems
3. develop short-term treatment objectives
4. develop reliable and valid data collection procedures to document progress over time
5. define the treatment program
6. analyze the results

These procedures were piloted on six subjects to assure their usefulness. These children received therapy twice a week for eight weeks. Their case profiles are presented in Appendix A.

A case study research design is most suitable for studying the efficacy of interventions for several reasons:

1. Children with motor impairments are a heterogenous group, and typically exhibit a wide range of associated handicaps, which makes pooling subjects difficult.

2. The treatments used are individualized; a standard treatment regime cannot be applied to all subjects. Each child's program is drawn from a collection of handling techniques and management strategies.

3. A case study design lends itself to the use of individualized assessment procedures that are sensitive to the specific needs of individuals with motor handicaps.

What Are the Research Questions?

Some of the research questions that may be answered by using the methods described in this section include:

1. How do children with motor impairments change when they receive short-term intervention?

   — Are the changes reflected in qualitative motor performance?

   — Are there other areas of development that improve as a result of the total therapy and educational management program (e.g., play, sensory processing)?

   — Does the child demonstrate overall improvement in the areas measured?

2. What are the specific treatment techniques and components of the management program that contribute to change?

3. What other variables (besides the specific intervention studied) might affect the child's progress (e.g., maturity, surgery)?

Steps in Documenting Progress

Step 1. Describe the child receiving treatment. First, obtain information about the child's history and performance level. The child's history should include information about the child's prenatal and neonatal history, medical history, and developmental course over time. Good records should be kept of educational or therapy programs in which the child participates. The use of orthotics should be documented as well.

Since children with motor impairments are a heterogeneous group, it is important to describe the child's developmental status. A developmental screening test should be administered to provide an overall baseline about the child's cognitive, language, motor, and social-emotional abilities. There are a number of developmental assessment tools that may be used to screen the child's overall developmental abilities. Many of these are described in detail in *A Therapist's Guide to Pediatric Assessment* (Stowers and Huber 1987). Some screening tools that are often used include the *Denver Developmental Screening Test* (Frankenburg et al. 1975), the *Miller Assessment for Preschoolers* (Miller 1982), the *Gesell Preschool Test* (Ames et al. 1980), the *Vineland Adaptive Behavior Scales* (Sparrow, Balla, and Cicchetti 1984), *Learning Accomplishment Profile-Diagnostic* (LeMay et al. 1977), the *Learning Accomplishment Profile-Revised* (Sanford and Zelman 1981), and the *Vulpe Assessment Battery* (Vulpe 1977).

Step 2. Measuring the child's primary problems. Refer to Part II of this manual for details on how to measure the child's primary problems.

Step 3. Collecting data about how the child responds to therapy.

The Pre- and Post-Test. If at all possible, it is very useful to videotape the assessments that are administered before and after the treatment intervention program. The same materials and methods of testing should be used for each. What is done during the videotape observations will differ for each child. Refer to Part II to determine what you might do for the pre- and post-test. After the pre-test, the child's primary problems should be identified. These will directly relate to the therapy or the educational short-term objectives.

When using the pre-test for research: The assessments should be scored by two unbiased independent evaluators. Observations to be made by each evaluator should be discussed prior to rating the videotape observations. Observations should be made independently of one another, listing primary problems that were observed. The evaluators may confer to discuss how they agree or differ in their observations. When there is a marked discrepancy in their agreement of the child's primary problems, another evaluator should observe the videotape. The third observer's findings will "settle" the difference. This procedure will provide a reliability check in determining the child's primary problems. Reliability should be calculated based on the following formula:

$$\text{Percent of Agreement} = \text{Agreements} \times 100 / \text{Agreements} + \text{Disagreements}$$

Step 4. Defining the treatment program. The next important step is to define the treatment procedures. This is done by describing the treatment that was provided. At least two therapy sessions should be videotaped over the course of the therapy program that the therapist feels are representative of the treatment provided. When conducting research, a panel of experts, that is, therapists skilled in the use of NDT, should observe the videotapes and independently describe what was done and why. There should be at least two therapists on the panel who take detailed notes about the types of therapy techniques used by the treating therapist and why those techniques were used. Agreement should be reached between the panel of experts on what treatment techniques were actually used and for what purpose. This provides a "fidelity" check in defining the therapy program. By describing the treatment provided, the specific areas addressed by the therapy program can be identified.

A more general way to define the therapy process is by documenting the variables that impact the therapy provided (e.g., setting, frequency and length of treatment, types of handling techniques used, parent involvement). For example, how much of the therapy session was direct hands-on, and how much involved parent training? Did the therapist use toys to motivate the child to move? Was mobile equipment used? Was NDT combined with other types of handling techniques? Was sensory integrative therapy used? Many variables affect an intervention program and need to be documented.

Step 5. Analyzing the results. There are three primary ways to analyze the results of the treatment program:

1. Comparison of pre- and post-test scores on the assessment measures

2. Inspection of data for trends in qualitative and quantitative performance, as indicated on the therapist and parent daily log sheets

3. Descriptive information provided in the parent interview regarding positive changes as a result of treatment

Note: Most of the analyses described herein are nonparametric data analyses because the data are ordinal, not comparative, in nature.

a. *Difference between pre- and post-test measures.* The pre- and post test changes from the child assessment measures can be calculated by noting differences in performance levels on the various evaluations administered. The differences in pre- and post-test assessments will serve to quantify functional and qualitative changes. They should be validated by descriptive information provided in the parent interview.

For our case example, John, the changes that were reflected on the assessment measures included the following:

- cruises at furniture

- squats in play

- stands momentarily

- holds small objects with tips of fingers instead of palm

- pulls off shirt over the head

- purposeful use of gestures

- follows simple directions

- plays independently and explores environment on his own

John was not performing any of the above skills prior to the eight-week intervention program. As this list makes apparent, qualitative changes in performance were not necessarily noted. For example, what was the quality of his cruising? Did some of the qualitative problems that were noted during the assessment (e.g., leans into furniture when standing) improve as well? In the next section, these types of observations are analyzed.

b. *Changes documented by the therapy logs.* Behaviors on the therapist and parent daily log sheets are coded for the presence or absence of skills. To do this make up a grid from session 1 through the last session. Then list the behaviors that were measured and check off with a "+" for observed and "–" for not present. You can then look at how the child performs over time and ask the following questions:

1. Did the skill show stability over time?

2. Was there a trend for improvement of the skill over time?

3. Was there overall improvement for all of the behaviors that were observed?

For individuals interested in research or calculating whether there was a significant difference in how the child performed, the following analyses may be conducted:

1. *Analysis of stability*

Select one behavior that was measured by the therapist or by the parent in the daily observation log sheets. List whether or not the child performed the skill each session, indicating with a "+" for presence or a "–" for absence of the skill.

Example: One of the behaviors measured by the therapist was whether or not John, while sitting on a therapy bench, could reach behind his body to obtain a toy, a skill that required thoracic extension, humeral external rotation, and neck and upper body rotation. The data collected by the therapist is presented in table B.1.

In this particular example, it is apparent that John developed the skill quite quickly after intervention was directed toward this problem.

2. *Analysis of trends*

There are two questions that we want to ask when analyzing trends:

- Did the child show improvement in specific behaviors observed over time;

- Was there overall improvement across all of the behaviors measured?

Calculate the number of positive and negative signs for a given skill for the first, second, third, and fourth quarters of the treatment program.

TABLE B.1
Observations of Reach in Sitting for Clinical Case: John

Session #	Presence or absence of skill
1	−
2	+
3	+
4	−
5	+
6	+
7	+
8	+
9	+
10	+
11	+
12	+
13	+
14	+
15	+
16	+

In our example of John, let's calculate his overall improvement across all of the measures obtained by the therapist. His results are presented in table B.2.

TABLE B.2
Overall Improvement: John

	Quarter				
	1st	2nd	3rd	4th	Total
Positive responses	31	34	39	40	144
Negative responses	9	6	1	0	16
	40	40	40	40	160

3. *Description of results*

A summary of major impressions about the results should be written. First write a brief, general statement about the treatment objective and the trends observed over the course of the treatment program. Describe the change in relation to the treatment objectives.

In our example, John demonstrated continual improvement in skills from the first through the fourth quarters of treatment. Most of his improvement was in the first 75% of the treatment program, which suggests that new observations were needed by the end of the eight-week treatment session for the "next-step" goals. When we look at the specific observations conducted by the therapist, the same trend holds. When we inspect the changes that occurred for the parent measures, there was improvement over time for all skills except fine motor skills involving reach, grasp, and release (e.g., pulling the string toy, opening the door, and building the two-cube tower). However, those fine motor skills for which John manipulated objects against a stable surface (e.g., scribbles, puts cup down without spilling, and stirring with a spoon) showed improvement.

Summary

This section describes methods for describing subjects, data collection, documentation of treatment, and data analyses. The reader is referred to books that detail single-subject research design for additional information about research design and statistical analyses (Bailey 1991; Royeen 1989; Tawney and Gast 1989). The case profiles presented in Appendix A should be examined in detail to assist in interpreting data.

Appendix C

REPRODUCIBLE LOG SHEETS AND SAMPLES

Directions for Using the Reproducible Log Sheets

Step 1. Using **Log Sheet 1,** list the problems or concerns that you feel should be the focus of the intervention program for the child over the next three months. Interview the parents to discover their greatest concerns, and to find out their preferred focus of intervention for the next three months.

Step 2. Referring to the problem/concern list that you and the parents generate (Log Sheet 1), think of specific observations that you could make during or immediately after an intervention session that would assess progress in these areas. Use the top section of **Log Sheet 2** for this purpose. These observations should be quick and easy to score.

Step 3. Drawing upon the parents' list of concerns, discuss together some things that would be reasonable and easy for them to observe of their child's behavior at home, if they choose to do this. Be sure that the parents understand what each of the observations mean. These observations should be very easy to do. List the observations that the parents agree to make on the bottom section of Log Sheet 2.

Step 4. Using the measures you have compiled on Log Sheet 2, fill out on **Log Sheet 3** the specific skills the therapist or educator will observe. Do the same on **Log Sheet 4** for observations the parents will make. Then photocopy a supply of these logs. Parents and therapist will use them over the next few months of intervention to record what they observe. Whoever is making observations of the child at least once a week—therapist, educator, parents—should be given a supply for ready use.

Step 5. The therapist, educator, and parents should make regular observations on the sheets at least once a week. Ideally, observations should be made twice a week. Simply check off whether the child completed the skill or not. If the skill was not observed, indicate that in the appropriate box.

Step 6. The log sheets should be collected from the parents every two weeks or so, and reviewed to determine how the child is progressing in the home environment. If the observations are too difficult for the parents to make, simplify the directions so that they are easier to follow—and so that you can still collect meaningful information from this source. Some parents may decide not to participate in this aspect of record keeping.

Step 7. After the child has participated in 16 observations spanning the course of about eight weeks, evaluate how the child performed over time for each skill. Make photocopies of **Log Sheet 5** for each of the skills that were observed by the therapist, educator, and parents. At the top of each sheet, fill in which skill was observed and how you determined whether or not the child completed it. This information is taken from Log Sheets 2, 3, and 4. Put a "+" in the box if the skill was completed, and a "-" in the box if the skill was not completed on that particular observation day. After completing this form, you will be able to tell whether:

1. A skill is only sometimes present and is not consolidated (e.g., more "-"s than "+"s);

2. A skill is emerging (e.g., more "+"s than "-"s);

3. A skill is developed and is consistently present (e.g., majority of "+"s).

Log Sheet 1   *Problem/Concern List*

Child's name: *Taprice*   Age: *15 mos.* Date: _____

Primary presenting problems:

List the main problems that should be a focus of therapy for the child in the next three months.

1. Stiffness in right arm, trunk, and both lower extremities
2. Limited use of right arm and hand
3. Predominance of asymmetrical tonic neck reflex in supine
4. Unable to roll from back to stomach and reach for feet in supine
5. Unable to weight shift in prone while prone on elbows
6. Poor head control in supported sitting

Parents' concerns:

List the things that the parents are most concerned about for their child and that they would like addressed by the intervention program for the next three months.

1. Unable to occupy herself with toys; needs adults to help constantly
2. Unable to hold objects in right hand
3. Difficult to bathe and dress because of weak head control
4. No interest in exploring environment
5.
6.

Log Sheet 2 · *Observation List*

Child's name: *Taprice*   Age: *15 mos.* Date: _____

Measures to Be Completed by Therapist or Educator at End of Intervention Session:

Using the primary presenting problems and concern list from the parents, list specific observations that could be made during or after intervention has been provided on a given day. Observations should be quick and easy to score.

1. Brings hands to midline and reaches for knees or feet while backlying
2. Reaches with right hand while backlying or in supported sitting
3. Keeps head centered while on back and can turn head to either side without ATNR
4. Rolls from back to stomach
5. Props in prone and weight shifts to reach for toy
6. Holds and shakes rattle in right hand
7. Holds head steady in supported sitting for 3 minutes

Observations that Parents Would Like to Make at Home Once or Twice a Week:

Using the problem/concern lists, discuss with the parents some things that they could observe at home about their child, if they so choose. The observations should be very easy to make.

1. After positioned in sidelying or in corner chair, Taprice plays with toys by herself for 5 minutes
2. Holds rattle or similar toy in right hand
3. Holds head up steadily for several minutes during bath or dressing
4. Taprice looks around room and shows interest in toys and people
5. _____
6. _____

Log Sheet 3

Therapist/Educator Worksheet

Child's name: *Taprice* _____ Age: *15 mos* Date: _____

Directions: Fill out a listing of skills to be observed during or after the intervention session. Simply check off if the skill was completed or not completed. If it was not observed on that particular day, indicate with a "N/O." Photocopy enough copies of the form for use over the next few months.

Skills	Completed	Not completed	Not observed
1. Hands to midline in supine			
2. Reaches for knees or feet in supine			
3. Reaches with right hand in supine or sit			
4. Keeps head centered while backlying			
5. Turns head to either side in supine without ATNR			
6. Rolls from back to stomach			
7. Props in prone; weight shifts to reach for toy			
8. Shakes rattle held in right hand			
9. Holds head steady in supported sitting for 3 minutes			
10.			

Log Sheet 4   *Parent Worksheet*

Child's name: *Taprice*   Age: *15 mos* Date: _____

Directions: After a therapist (or teacher) has discussed your personal concerns for your child with you, a checklist will be developed of some skills to observe in your child at home. Your therapist will give you a number of copies of this form for your use over the next few months. Pick two times of the week that are convenient for you to observe these skills. Simply check off in the "completed" or "not completed" boxes whether or not your child was able to do the skill. If you were not able to observe the skill, then check off "not observed." Take the completed copies to your child's therapist (or teacher) every two weeks. The therapist will see what you are noticing about your child. This feedback is very important, because it allows the therapist to understand how your child is progressing at home.

Skills	Completed	Not completed	Not observed
1. *Plays with toys by herself for 5 min.*			
2. *Holds rattle or toy in right hand*			
3. *Holds head steady for several minutes when being dressed or bathed*			
4. *Shows interest in moving, reaching, and interacting with toys and people*			
5.			
6.			
7.			
8.			
9.			
10.			

Log Sheet 5   *Skill Evaluation*

Child's name: *Taprice*

Skill observed: *Hands to midline in supine*

Criterion for completing skill: *While backlying, Taprice brings both hands to midline to touch toy or to touch other hand*

Skill Completion

Session	1	2	3	4	5	6	7	8	9	10	11	12	13	14	15	16
Skill completed? (Indicate with "+" for yes and "-" for no)	−	+	−	−	+	−	−	+	+	−	−	−	+	+	−	+

Log Sheet 5   *Skill Evaluation*

Child's name: *Taprice*

Skill observed: *Reaches for knees or feet*

Criterion for completing skill: *While backlying, Taprice reaches for her knees or feet, showing anti-gravity flexion*

Skill Completion

Session	1	2	3	4	5	6	7	8	9	10	11	12	13	14	15	16
Skill completed? (Indicate with "+" for yes and "-" for no)	−	−	−	−	−	−	+	−	+	−	−	+	+	−	+	+

Log Sheet 5   *Skill Evaluation*

Child's name: *Taprice*

Skill observed: *Reaches with right hand*

Criterion for completing skill: *While supine or in supported sitting, Taprice reaches for toy held in space with her right hand*

Skill Completion

Session	1	2	3	4	5	6	7	8	9	10	11	12	13	14	15	16
Skill completed? (Indicate with "+" for yes and "-" for no)	−	−	−	−	−	−	+	+	−	+	+	+	−	+	+	+

Log Sheet 5   *Skill Evaluation*

Child's name: *Taprice*

Skill observed: *Keeps head centered while backlying*

Criterion for completing skill: *Head remains steady and centered in supine at least 80% time observed (2-minute observation)*

Skill Completion

Session	1	2	3	4	5	6	7	8	9	10	11	12	13	14	15	16
Skill completed? (Indicate with "+" for yes and "-" for no)	−	−	−	−	+	−	−	+	−	+	+	−	+	+	+	+

Log Sheet 5   *Skill Evaluation*

Child's name: *Taprice*

Skill observed: *Turns head in supine without ATNR*

Criterion for completing skill: *While backlying, turns head freely to either side to look at toy without showing ATNR*

Skill Completion

Session	1	2	3	4	5	6	7	8	9	10	11	12	13	14	15	16
Skill completed? (Indicate with "+" for yes and "-" for no)	−	−	+	−	−	−	−	+	−	−	+	+	−	+	+	+

Log Sheet 5   *Skill Evaluation*

Child's name: *Taprice*

Skill observed: *Rolls from back to stomach*

Criterion for completing skill: *When encouraged, rolls within 1 minute from back to stomach toward the left or right side*

Skill Completion

Session	1	2	3	4	5	6	7	8	9	10	11	12	13	14	15	16
Skill completed? (Indicate with "+" for yes and "-" for no)	−	−	−	+	−	+	−	−	+	+	+	+	+	+	+	+

Log Sheet 5   *Skill Evaluation*

Child's name: *Taprice*

Skill observed: *Props in prone; weight shifts to reach for toy*

Criterion for completing skill: *When placed in prone, will shift weight onto one arm to reach for toy placed in front of body*

Skill Completion

Session	1	2	3	4	5	6	7	8	9	10	11	12	13	14	15	16
Skill completed? (Indicate with "+" for yes and "-" for no)	+	-	-	+	-	-	+	+	-	+	+	-	+	+	+	+

Log Sheet 5   *Skill Evaluation*

Child's name: *Taprice*

Skill observed: *Shakes rattle held in right hand*

Criterion for completing skill: *When rattle is placed in right hand, Taprice shakes it, retaining her grasp for at least 1 minute*

Skill Completion

Session	1	2	3	4	5	6	7	8	9	10	11	12	13	14	15	16
Skill completed? (Indicate with "+" for yes and "-" for no)	+	-	-	+	+	-	+	+	+	+	-	+	+	+	+	+

Log Sheet 5 — *Skill Evaluation*

Child's name: *Taprice*

Skill observed: *Holds head steady in supported sitting*

Criterion for completing skill: *When placed in supported sitting, holding Taprice at her pelvis, she holds her head steady 3 minutes*

Skill Completion

Session	1	2	3	4	5	6	7	8	9	10	11	12	13	14	15	16
Skill completed? (Indicate with "+" for yes and "-" for no)	−	−	−	−	+	−	+	+	−	+	+	+	+	+	+	+

Log Sheet 5 — *Skill Evaluation*

Child's name: *Taprice*

Skill observed: *Plays with toys by herself for 5 minutes*

Criterion for completing skill: *When placed on the floor or in her corner chair, Taprice plays with interesting toys: looking, touching, and holding them*

Skill Completion

Session	1	2	3	4	5	6	7	8	9	10	11	12	13	14	15	16
Skill completed? (Indicate with "+" for yes and "-" for no)	−	−	−	+	−	+	+	−	+	+	+	+	+	+	+	+

Log Sheet 5 *Skill Evaluation*

Child's name: *Taprice*

Skill observed: *Shows interest in moving, reaching, and interacting with toys and people*

Criterion for completing skill: *When toys and people are near her, Taprice looks, vocalizes, reaches, smiles, or tries to move toward them in a 5-minute observation*

Skill Completion

Session	1	2	3	4	5	6	7	8	9	10	11	12	13	14	15	16
Skill completed? (Indicate with "+" for yes and "-" for no)	−	−	−	+	−	+	−	+	+	+	+	+	+	+	+	+

Child's name: _____ Age: _____ Date: _____

Primary presenting problems:

List the main problems that should be a focus of therapy for the child in the next three months.

1. _____
   _____

2. _____
   _____

3. _____
   _____

4. _____
   _____

5. _____
   _____

6. _____
   _____

Parents' concerns:

List the things that the parents are most concerned about for their child and that they would like addressed by the intervention program for the next three months.

1. _____
   _____

2. _____
   _____

3. _____
   _____

4. _____
   _____

5. _____
   _____

6. _____
   _____

Log Sheet 2   *Observation List*

Child's name: _____ Age: _____ Date: _____

Measures to Be Completed by Therapist or Educator at End of Intervention Session:

Using the primary presenting problems and concern list from the parents, list specific observations that could be made during or after intervention has been provided on a given day. Observations should be quick and easy to score.

1. _____

   _____

2. _____

   _____

3. _____

   _____

4. _____

   _____

5. _____

   _____

6. _____

   _____

Observations that Parents Would Like to Make at Home Once or Twice a Week:

Using the problem/concern lists, discuss with the parents some things that they could observe at home about their child, if they so choose. The observations should be very easy to make.

1. _____

   _____

2. _____

   _____

3. _____

   _____

4. _____

   _____

5. _____

   _____

6. _____

   _____

Log Sheet 3

Therapist/Educator Worksheet

Child's name: _____ Age: _____ Date: _____

Directions: Fill out a listing of skills to be observed during or after the intervention session. Simply check off if the skill was completed or not com- pleted. If it was not observed on that particular day, indicate with a "N/O." Photocopy enough copies of the form for use over the next few months.

Skills	Completed	Not completed	Not observed
1. _____			
2. _____			
3. _____			
4. _____			
5. _____			
6. _____			
7. _____			
8. _____			
9. _____			
10. _____			

Child's name: _____ Age: _____ Date: _____

Directions: After a therapist (or teacher) has discussed your personal concerns for your child with you, a checklist will be developed of some skills to observe in your child at home. Your therapist will give you a number of copies of this form for your use over the next few months. Pick two times of the week that are convenient for you to observe these skills. Simply check off in the "completed" or "not completed" boxes whether or not your child was able to do the skill. If you were not able to observe the skill, then check off "not observed." Take the completed copies to your child's therapist (or teacher) every two weeks. The therapist will see what you are noticing about your child. This feedback is very important, because it allows the therapist to understand how your child is progressing at home.

Skills	Completed	Not completed	Not observed
1. _____			
2. _____			
3. _____			
4. _____			
5. _____			
6. _____			
7. _____			
8. _____			
9. _____			
10. _____			

Child's name: _____

Skill observed: _____

Criterion for completing skill: _____

_____

Skill Completion

Session	1	2	3	4	5	6	7	8	9	10	11	12	13	14	15	16
Skill completed? (Indicate with "+" for yes and "–" for no)																

Log Sheet 5   *Skill Evaluation*

Child's name: _____

Skill observed: _____

Criterion for completing skill: _____

_____

Skill Completion

Session	1	2	3	4	5	6	7	8	9	10	11	12	13	14	15	16
Skill completed? (Indicate with "+" for yes and "–" for no)																

Glossary

Arousal—A basic alerting mechanism allowing for transition from sleep to a wakeful state; necessary for attention; relates to basic sensory registration.

Attention—Involves arousal and alerting, habituation and interest in novelty, capacity to sustain effort, selection and screening of stimuli, and motivation and persistence to stay on-task.

Attentional deficit—Cluster of symptoms, including distractibility, poor concentration, lack of persistence, poor self-monitoring, disorganization, and impulsivity.

Cocontraction—The simultaneous contraction of agonist and antagonist muscles.

Communication—The intentional signalling of meanings to others using gestures, words, or other behaviors.

Defensiveness—A severe sensitivity to sensory stimulation; adverse reaction to experiences not normally considered noxious.

Effectiveness—In research, this refers to the relative benefits of one intervention over another.

Efficacy—In research, this refers to gains or benefits obtained over time when an intervention is provided.

Emotion regulation—The mediating influence of emotions on behavior; the capacity to organize emotions into meaningful life experiences.

Equilibrium reaction—The compensatory movements of the trunk and limbs to regain midline alignment and stability when center of gravity is displaced.

Facilitation—The provision of carefully selected sensory stimulation and/or guiding of movement to produce an adaptive sensorimotor response.

Functional performance—The drive or motivation to engage in purposeful activity, and the capacity to adapt to environmental demands.

Gravitational insecurity—An extreme fearfulness in moving in space, with strong preference for close-to-ground body positions.

Holistic—Meaning to encompass a wide range of behaviors, domains, or processes.

Homeostasis—A basic engagement and interest in the world that relates to physiological maturation, caregiver responsivity, and adaptation to environmental demands.

Hypersensitivity—An increased sensitivity to sensory stimulation with adverse reaction.

Hypertonicity—A stiffness or spasticity in muscles; too much tension or resistance in muscles to passive movement.

Hyposensitivity—A decreased sensory awareness or under-responsiveness to sensory stimulation.

Hypotonicity—A flaccidity in muscles with lack of resistance; floppiness in movement quality.

Inhibition—The prevention or interruption of abnormal movement and postural responses.

Motor control—Mechanisms that allow an individual to regulate and coordinate motor actions to perform a task.

Motor learning—Mechanisms by which skilled movements are acquired.

Motor planning (praxis)—The ability to conceptualize and automatically organize and plan sequential movements in time and space.

Muscle tone—The elasticity of muscle; ability of muscle to tense in different positions; a condition of readiness to move.

Neurodevelopmental—The focus on adaptive movement and postural responses during functional living skills.

Neuromotor handicap—Abnormal muscle tone, delayed reflex maturation, poor movement quality, and delay in functional motor skills.

Play—The wide range of behaviors that comprise relationships with other persons, objects, events, and situations.

Postural responses—Righting and equilibrium reactions that underlie automatic movement.

Postural control—The capacity to hold the body in stable positions against gravity to allow for functional movement.

Postural tone—Postural adjustments that allow the child to move against gravity and to attain a variety of movement patterns; redistributions in muscle tone in response to changes in body position, alignment, or shifts in center of gravity.

Primitive reflexes—The phasic and tonic reflexes present at birth.

Proprioception—The reception of information from muscles, tendons, and joints, leading to an internal awareness of body parts and their position in space.

Reductionistic—The examination of individual performance in discrete, fine-grained analysis.

Representational meanings—The abstraction of functional meaning of human and inanimate objects, events, and situations.

Righting reactions—Automatic body reactions that return the body midline into alignment with the center of gravity.

Reflexes—Simple, predictable body responses or movements resulting from sensory stimulation.

Reflex maturation—The development of normal automatic righting and equilibrium reactions.

Release phenomenon—The hypothesized activation of abnormal reflex activity as a result of poor cortical inhibition.

Self-care—Refers to daily living tasks, including feeding, dressing, hygiene, and other everyday life skills.

Sensory processing—The integration and synthesis of sensory stimulation to allow for a purposeful, goal-directed response.

Somatosensory—The sensation of touch perceived by the skin and including receptors that perceive pain, temperature, light touch, pressure, and vibration.

Tactile—Sensory stimulation perceived through the skin. It involves general awareness of the environment through the sense of touch, temperature, and pain.

Tonal disturbance—A disturbance in muscle or postural tone affecting coordination and movement.

Tone (muscle)—Related to the degrees of tension present in the resting state of a muscle.

Vestibular—An inner ear mechanism that perceives body movement in space and is important for maintaining plane of vision in response to movement, balance, and security in movement.

References

Abidin, R. R. 1986. *Parenting stress index*. Charlottesville, VA: Pediatric Psychology Press.

Achenbach, T. M. 1989. *Child behavior checklist*. Burlington, VT: University of Vermont.

Ames, L. B., C. Gillespie, J. Haines, and F. L. Ilg. 1980. *Gesell preschool test for evaluating motor, adaptive, language, and personal-social behavior in children ages 2¹/₂-6*. New Haven, CT: Programs for Education, Inc.

Amiel-Tison, C., and A. Grenier. 1983. *Neurologic evaluation of the newborn and the infant*. New York: Masson Publishing USA.

Andre-Thomas, de Ajuriaguerra J., Y. Chesni, and S. Saint-Anne Dargassies. 1960. *The neurological examination of the infant*. Little Club Clinics in Developmental Medicine, No. 1. London: National Spastics Society.

Ayres, A. J. 1972. *Sensory integration and learning disorders*. Los Angeles: Western Psychological Services.

_____. "Sensorimotor Foundations of Academic Ability." In *Perceptual and learning disabilities in children*, vol. 2, edited by W. M. Cruickshank and D. P. Hallahan, 301-360. Syracuse, NY: Syracuse University Press, 1975.

_____. 1979. *Sensory integration and the child*. Los Angeles: Western Psychological Services.

_____. 1985. *Developmental dyspraxia and adult onset apraxia*. Torrance, CA: Sensory Integration International.

_____. 1989. *Sensory Integration and Praxis Tasks*. Los Angeles: Western Psychological Services.

Ayres, A. J., and L. S. Tickle. 1980. Hyper-responsivity to touch and vestibular stimuli as a predictor of positive response to sensory integration procedures by autistic children. *American Journal of Occupational Therapy* 34:375-81.

Bailey, D. M. 1991. *Research for the health professional: A practical guide.* Philadelphia: F. A. Davis, Co.

Bauer, B. A. 1977. Tactile-sensitive behavior in hyperactive and nonhyperactive children. *American Journal of Occupational Therapy* 31:447-53.

Bayley, N. 1969. *Bayley scales of infant development.* New York: Psychological Corporation.

Bettelheim, B. 1987. The importance of play. *Atlantic Monthly.* March:35-46.

Bly, L. 1983. *Components of normal movement during the first year of life.* Chicago: Neuro-Developmental Treatment Association, Inc.

Bobath, B. 1959. The neuropathy of cerebral palsy and its importance in treatment and diagnosis. *Cerebral Palsy Bulletin* 1:13-33.

_____. 1985. *Abnormal postural reflex activity caused by brain lesions,* 3d ed. Rockville, MD: Aspen Publications.

Bobath, K. 1971. The normal postural reflex mechanism and its deviation in children with cerebral palsy. *Physiotherapy* 57:515-25.

Bobath, K., and B. Bobath. 1952. A treatment of cerebral palsy based on the analysis of the patient's motor behavior. *British Journal of Physical Medicine* 15:107-17.

_____. 1956. The diagnosis of cerebral palsy in infancy. *Archives of Disease in Childhood* 31(159):408-14.

_____. 1964. The facilitation of normal postural reactions and movements in the treatment of cerebral palsy. *Physiotherapy* 50:246-62.

_____. 1984. "Neuro-Developmental Treatment." In *Management of the Motor Disorders in the Children with Cerebral Palsy,* edited by D. Scrutton, Philadelphia: J. B. Lippencott

Bornstein, M. H., and M. D. Sigman. 1986. Continuity in mental development from infancy. *Child Development* 57:251-74.

Brazelton, T. B. 1984. *Neonatal behavioral assessment scale,* 2d ed. Clinics in Developmental Medicine, No. 88. Philadelphia: J. B. Lippincott.

Brooks, V. 1986. *The neural basis of motor control.* New York: Oxford University Press.

Bzoch, K. R., and R. League. 1970. *Receptive-expressive emergent language scale.* Baltimore: University Park Press.

Capute, A., P. Accardo, E. Vining, J. Rubenstein, and S. Harryman. 1978. *Primitive reflex profile.* Baltimore: University Park Press.

Carey, W. B., and S. C. McDermitt. 1980. Minimal brain dysfunction and hyperkinesis. *American Journal of Disabled Children* 134:926-29

Carrow-Woolfolk, E. 1973. *Test of auditory comprehension of language (TACL)*. Hingham, MA: Teaching Resources Corporation.

Cermak, S. "Developmental Dyspraxia." In *Advances in psychology*. Vol. 23, *Neuropsychological studies of apraxia and related disorders,* edited by E. A. Roy, 225-248. New York: Elsevier Science Publishers, 1985.

Chandler, L., M. Andrews, M. Swanson, and A. Larson. 1987. *Chandler movement assessment of infants*. P.O. Box 4631, Rolling Bay, Washington.

Clark, D. L. 1985. The vestibular system: An overview of structure and function. *Physical and Occupational Therapy in Pediatrics* 5:5-32.

Cohen, H., and E. A. Keshner. 1989. Current concepts of the vestibular system reviewed: Part 2. Visual/vestibular interaction and spatial orientation. *American Journal of Occupational Therapy* 43(5):331-38.

Dargassies, S. S. A. 1972. Neurodevelopmental symptoms during the first year of life. *Developmental Medicine and Child Neurology* 14:235-46.

Davies, D. R., and R. Parasuraman. 1984. *Varieties of attention*. New York: Academic Press.

DeGangi, G. A., R. A. Berk, and J. Valvano. 1983. Test of motor and neurological functions in high-risk infants: Preliminary findings. *Developmental and Behavioral Pediatrics* 4(3):182-89.

DeGangi, G. A., R. A. Berk, and S. I. Greenspan. 1988. The clinical measurement of sensory functioning in infants: A preliminary study. *Physical and Occupational Therapy in Pediatrics* 8(2/3):1-23.

DeQuiros, J. 1976. Diagnosis of vestibular disorders in the learning disabled. *Journal of Learning Disabilities* 9(1):50-58.

Drillien, C. M. 1972. Abnormal neurological signs in the first year of life in low birth weight infants: Possible prognostic significance. *Developmental Medicine and Child Neurology* 14:575-84.

Drillien, C., A. Thomson, and K. Burgoyne. 1980. Low birthweight children at early school age: A longitudinal study. *Developmental Medicine and Child Neurology* 22:26-47.

Dunn, L. M., and L. M. Dunn. 1981. *Peabody Picture Vocabulary Test,* rev. ed. "(PVT-R) Forms L and M." Circle Pines, MN: American Guidance Services.

Ellenberg, J. H., and K. B. Nelson. 1981. Early recognition of infants at high risk for cerebral palsy: Examination at age four months. *Developmental Medicine and Child Neurology* 23:705-16.

Ellison, P. H., J. L. Horn, and C. A. Browning. 1985. Construction of an infant neurological international battery (INFANIB) for the assessment of neurological integrity in infancy. *Physical Therapy* 65(9):1326-31.

Fagan, J. F. 1982. New evidence for the prediction of intelligence from infancy. *Infant Mental Health Journal* 3(4):219-28.

Fisher, A. G., E. A. Murray, and A. C. Bundy, eds. *Sensory integration: Theory and practice.* Philadelphia: F. A. Davis Co., 1989.

Fisher, A. G., and A. C. Bundy. "Vestibular Stimulation in the Treatment of Postural and Related Disorders." In *Manual of physical therapy techniques,* edited by O. D. Payton, R. P. DiFabio, S. V. Paris, E. J. Protas, and A. F. VanSant, 239-258. New York: Churchill Livingstone, 1989.

Folio, R., and R. Fewell. 1983. *Peabody Developmental Motor Scales (PDMS).* Allen, TX: DLM Teaching Resources.

Frankenburg, W. K., et al. 1975. *Denver developmental screening test: Reference manual,* rev. ed. Denver: University of Colorado Medical Center.

Gilfoyle, E. M., A. P. Grady, and J. C. Moore. 1990. *Children adapt,* 2d ed. Thorofare, NJ: Slack, Inc.

Gordon, J. "Disorders of Motor Control." In *Key issues in neurological physiotherapy,* edited by L. Ada and C. Canning, 25-50. London: Heinemann, 1990.

Gorga, D. 1989. Occupational therapy treatment practices with infants in early intervention. *American Journal of Occupational Therapy* 43:731-35.

Greenberg, R., and T. Field. 1982. Temperament ratings of handicapped infants during classroom, mother and teacher interactions. *Journal of Pediatric Psychology* 7:387-405.

Greenspan, S. I. 1979. Intelligence and adaptation: An integration of psychoanalytic and piagetian developmental psychology. *Psychological Issues,* Monograph 47/48. New York: International Universities Press.

———. 1989. *The development of the ego: Implications for personality theory, psychopathology, and the psychotherapeutic process.* Madison, CT: International Universities Press.

Greenspan, S. I., and R. S. Lourie. 1981. Developmental structuralist approach to the classification of adaptive and pathologic personality organizations: Infancy and early childhood. *American Journal of Psychiatry* 138(6):725-35.

Greenspan, S. I., and S. W. Porges. 1984. Psychopathology in infancy and early childhood: Clinical perspectives on the organization of sensory and affective-thematic experience. *Child Development* 55:49-70.

Harris, S. R., S. M. Haley, W. L. Tada, M. W. Swanson. 1984. Reliability of observational measures of the Movement Assessment of Infants. *Physical Therapy* 64(4):472-76.

Hedrick, D. L., E. M. Prather, and A. R. Tobin. 1975. *Sequenced inventory of communication development (SICD)*. Seattle, WA: University of Washington Press.

Illingworth, R. S. 1966. The diagnosis of cerebral palsy in the first year of life. *Developmental Medicine and Child Neurology* 8:178-94.

Izard, C. E. 1971. *The face of emotion*. New York: Appleton-Century-Crofts.

Jelm, J. 1990. *Oral-motor/feeding rating scale*. Tucson, AZ: Therapy Skill Builders.

Jennings, K. D., R. D. Connors, C. E. Stegman, P. Sankaranarayan, and S. Mendolsohn. 1985. Mastery motivation in young preschoolers. *Journal of the Division of Early Childhood* 9(2):162-69.

Kathrein, J. E. 1990. Interrater reliability in the assessment of muscle tone of infants and children. *Physical and Occupational Therapy in Pediatrics* 10(1):27-41.

Keshner, E. A., and H. Cohen. 1989. Current concepts of the vestibular system reviewed: Part 1. The role of the vestibular spinal system in postural control. *American Journal of Occupational Therapy* 43(5):320-30.

Kielhofner, G., ed. 1985. *A model of human occupation: Theory and application*. Baltimore: Williams and Wilkins.

Kopp, C. B. 1982. Antecedents of self-regulation: A developmental perspective. *Developmental Psychology* 12(4):199-214.

_____. 1982. Antecedents of self-regulation: A developmental perspective. *Developmental Psychology* 18:199-214.

_____. "The Growth of Self-Regulation: Parents and Children." In *Perspectives in developmental psychology*, edited by N. Eisenberg, 34-55. New York: Wiley, 1987.

_____. 1989. Regulation of distress and negative emotions: A developmental view. *Developmental Psychology* 25:343-54.

Langley, M. B., and L. J. Lombardino, eds. 1991. *Neurodevelopmental strategies for managing communication disorders in children with severe motor dysfunction*. Austin, TX: Pro-Ed.

LeMay, D. W., P. M. Griffin, and A. R. Sanford. 1977. *Learning accomplishment profile-diagnostic edition: Examiner's manual*, rev. Winston-Salem, NC: Kaplan Press.

Lewis, M. "Social Development in Infancy and Early Childhood." In *Handbook of infant development*, edited by J. D. Osofsky, 419-493. New York: John Wiley and Sons, 1987.

Li, A. K. F. 1981. Play and the mentally retarded. *Mental Retardation* 19:121-26.

Linder, T. W. 1990. *Transdisciplinary play-based assessment*. Baltimore: Paul H. Brookes Publishing Co.

Marsden, C. D. 1982. The mysterious motor function of the basal ganglia. *Neurology* 32:514-39.

Matthews, P. B. C. 1988. Proprioceptors and their contribution to somatosensory mapping: Complex messages require complex processing. *Canadian Journal of Physiology and Pharmacology* 66:430-38.

McCarthy, D. 1972. *McCarthy scales of children's abilities.* New York: Psychological Corp.

Miller, L. J. 1982. *The Miller assessment for preschoolers: Manual.* Littleton, CO: The Foundation for Knowledge in Development.

_____. 1994. *Toddler and infant motor evaluation (TIME).* Tucson, AZ: Therapy Skill Builders.

Molnar, G., and S. V. Gordon. 1976. Cerebral palsy: Predictive value of selected clinical signs for early prognostication of motor function. *Archives of Physical Medicine Rehabilitation* 57:153-58.

Molnar, G. E., and L. T. Taft. 1977. Pediatric rehabilitation, part 1: Cerebral palsy and spinal cord injury. *Current Problems in Pediatrics* 7:3-55.

Montagu, A. 1978. *Touching: The human significance of the skin.* New York: Harper and Row.

Naunton, R., ed. 1975. *The vestibular system.* New York: Academic Press.

Ornitz, E. 1970. Vestibular dysfunction in schizophrenia and childhood autism. *Comparative Psychiatry* 11:159-73.

Ottenbacher, K. J. 1982. Vestibular processing dysfunction in children with severe emotional and behavioral disorders: A review. *Physical and Occupational Therapy in Pediatrics* 2(1):3-12.

Ottenbacher, K. J., Z. Biocca, G. DeCremer, M. Gevelinger, K. B. Jedlovec, and M. B. Johnson. 1986. Quantitative analysis of the effectiveness of pediatric therapy. *Physical Therapy* 66(7):1095-101.

Paine, R. S. 1964. The evolution of infantile postural reflexes in the presence of chronic brain syndromes. *Developmental Medicine and Child Neurology* 6:345-61.

_____. 1969. Early recognition of neuromotor disability in infants of low birthweight. *Developmental Medicine and Child Neurology* 11:455-59.

Palfrey, J. S., M. D. Levine, D. K. Walker, and M. Sullivan. 1985. The emergence of attention deficits in early childhood: A prospective study. *Developmental and Behavioral Pediatrics* 6:339-48.

Palisano, R. J. 1991. Research on the effectiveness of neurodevelopmental treatment. *Pediatric Physical Therapy* 3(3):143-48.

Parette, H. P., and J. J. Hourcade. 1984. A review of therapeutic intervention research on gross and fine motor progress in young children with cerebral palsy. *American Journal of Occupational Therapy* 38:462-68.

Parette, H. P., M. D. Hendricks, and S. L. Rock. 1991. Efficacy of therapeutic intervention intensity with infants and young children with cerebral palsy. *Infants and Young Children* 4(2):1-19.

Porges, S. W. 1984. Physiologic correlates of attention: A core process underlying learning disorders. *Pediatric Clinics of North America* 31:31-45.

Reilly, M., ed. 1974. *Play as exploratory learning.* Beverly Hills: Sage Publications.

Rose, S. A., and I. F. Wallace. 1985. Visual recognition memory: A predictor of later cognitive functioning in preterms. *Child Development* 56:843-52.

Rosenblith, J. F., and R. B. Anderson. 1968. Prognostic significance of discrepancies in muscle tension between upper and lower limbs. *Developmental Medicine and Child Neurology* 10:322-30.

Royeen, C. B. 1987. Test-retest reliability of a touch scale for tactile defensiveness. *Physical and Occupational Therapy in Pediatrics* 7(3):45-52.

_____. 1989. *Clinical research handbook.* Thorofare, NJ: Slack, Inc.

Ruff, H. A. 1986. Components of attention during infants' manipulative exploration. *Child Development* 57:105-14.

Rutter, M. 1982. Syndromes attributed to minimal brain dysfunction in childhood. *American Journal of Psychiatry* 139:21-33.

Sanford, A. R., and J. G. Zelman. 1981. *Learning accomplishment profile,* rev. ed. Winston-Salem, NC: Kaplan Press.

Scherzer, A., and I. Tscharnuter. 1982. *Early diagnosis and therapy in cerebral palsy.* New York: Marcel Dekker, Inc.

Schmidt, R. A. "Motor Learning Principles for Physical Therapy." In *Two step contemporary management of motor control problems,* edited by M. Lister, 49-64. Alexandria, VA: Foundation for Physical Therapy, 1991.

Simeonsson, R. J., D. H. Cooper, and A. P. Scheiner. 1982. A review and analysis of the effectiveness of early intervention programs. *Pediatrics* 69:635-41.

Sparrow, S., D. Balla, and D. Cicchetti. 1984. *Vineland adaptive behavior scales: Interview edition.* Circle Pines, MN: American Guidance Service.

Stern, F. M., and D. Gorga. 1988. Neurodevelopmental treatment (NDT): Therapeutic intervention and its efficacy. *Infants and Young Children* 1:22-32.

Stowers, S., and C. J. Huber. "Developmental and Screening Tests." In *A Therapist's guide to pediatric assessment,* edited by L. King-Thomas and B. J. Hacker, 43-142. Boston: Little, Brown, & Co. 1987.

Tawney, J. W., and D. L. Gast. 1989. *Single subject research in special education.* Columbus, OH: Charles E. Merrill Publishing Co.

Valvano, J., and G. A. DeGangi. 1986. Atypical posture and movement findings in high risk pre-term infants. *Physical and Occupational Therapy in Pediatrics* 6:71-81.

Vulpe, S. 1977. *Vulpe assessment battery,* 2d ed. Downsview, Ontario: National Institute on Mental Retardation.

Weissbluth, M. "Sleep-Loss Stress and Temperamental Difficultness: Psychobiological Processes and Practical Considerations." In *Temperament in childhood,* edited by G. A. Kohnstamm, J. E. Bates, and M. K. Rothbart, 357-376. New York: Wiley & Sons, 1989.

Recommended Reading

Anderson, S. "Daily Care." In *Children with cerebral palsy,* edited by E. Geralis, 91-132. Kensington, MD: Woodbine House, 1991.

Ayres, A. J., Z. K. Mailloux, and C. L. Wendler. 1987. Developmental dyspraxia: Is it a unitary function? *Occupational Therapy Journal of Research* 7(2):93-110.

Berlyne, D. B. 1960. *Conflict, arousal, and curiosity.* New York: McGraw-Hill.

_____. 1965. *Structure and direction in thinking.* New York: Wiley & Sons.

Bly, L. 1983. *The components of normal movement during the first year of life and abnormal motor development.* Birmingham, AL: Pittenger & Associates.

Brazelton, T., B. Koslowski, and M. Main. "The Origins of Reciprocity: The Early Mother-Infant Interaction." In *The effect of the infant on its caregiver,* edited by M. Lewis and L. Rosenblum, 49-76. New York: Wiley & Sons, 1974.

Campbell, P. H., and B. Stewart. 1986. Measuring changes in movement skills with infants and young children with handicaps. *Journal of the Association for Persons with Severe Handicaps* 11(3):153-61.

Cohen, L. B. 1972. Attention-getting and attention holding processes of infant visual preferences. *Child Development* 43:869-79.

_____. "Habituation of Infant Visual Attention." In *Habituation: Perspectives from child development, animal behavior, and neurophysiology,* edited by T. J. Tighe and R. N. Leaton. Hillsdale, NJ: Lawrence Erlbaum Associates, 1976.

Conrad, K., S. A. Cermak, and C. Drake. 1983. Differentiation of praxis among children. *American Journal of Occupational Therapy* 37(7):466-73.

Dargassies, S. S. A. 1972. Neurodevelopmental symptoms during the first year of life. *Developmental Medicine and Child Neurology* 14:235-46.

Davies, D. R., and R. Parasuraman. 1984. *Varieties of attention*. New York: Academic Press.

DeGangi, G. A. 1991. Assessment of sensory, emotional, and attentional problems in regulatory disordered infants. *Infants and Young Children* 3(3):1-8.

DeGangi, G. A., L. Hurley, and T. R. Linscheid. 1983. Toward a methodology of the short-term effects of neurodevelopmental treatment. *American Journal of Occupational Therapy* 37(7):479-84.

DeGangi, G. A., and R. A. Berk. 1983. Assessment of sensory integrative dysfunction in the preschool years. *Learning Disabilities* 2(1):1-15.

DeGangi, G. A., and S. I. Greenspan. 1988. The development of sensory functions in infants. *Physical and Occupational Therapy in Pediatrics* 8(3):21-33.

Drillien, C. M. "Minor Abnormal Neurological Signs in the First Two Years of Life." In *Neurodevelopmental Problems in Early Childhood,* edited by C. M. Drillien and M. B. Drumond, 340-347. Oxford, England: Blackwell Scientific Publishers, 1977.

Dubowitz, L. M. S., Z. Dubowitz, P. G. Palmer, et al. 1984. Correlation of neurologic assessment in the preterm newborn infant with outcome at one year. *Journal of Pediatrics* 105:452-56.

Finnie, N. R. 1975. *Handling the Young Cerebral Palsied Child at Home,* 2d ed. New York: E. P. Dutton.

Fiorention, M. 1973. *Reflex testing methods for evaluating C.N.S. development.* Springfield, IL: Charles C. Thomas.

Gianino, A., and E. Z. Tronick. "The Mutual Regulation model: The Infant's Self and Interactive Regulation Coping and Defense." In *Stress and coping,* edited by T. Field, P. McCabe, and N. Schneiderman, 47-68. Hillsdale, NJ: Lawrence Erlbaum Associates, 1988.

Hanzlik, J. R. 1989. The effects of intervention on the free-play experience for mothers and their infants with developmental delay and cerebral palsy. *Physical and Occupational Therapy in Pediatrics* 9(2):33-51.

Harris, M. B., C. A. Dedrick, M. B. Downey, E. A. Long, and K. Persell-Beckett. 1985. A photographic method for the documentation of neuromotor problems and effects of treatment. *Physical and Occupational Therapy in Pediatrics* 6(1):75-91.

Hoskins, T. A., and J. E. Squires. 1973. Developmental assessment: A test for gross motor and reflex development. *Physical Therapy* 53:117-26.

Illingworth, R. S. 1966. The diagnosis of cerebral palsy in the first year of life. *Developmental Medicine and Child Neurology* 8:178-94.

———. 1961. Early diagnosis of cerebral palsy. *Medical World News* 94:218-20.

———. "Early Diagnosis and Differential Diagnosis." In *Recent advances in cerebral palsy,* edited by R. S. Illingworth. Boston: Little, Brown & Co., 1958.

James, W. 1884. What is an emotion? *Mind* 9:188-205.

Kahneman, D. 1973. *Attention and effort.* Englewood Cliffs, NJ: Prentice-Hall.

Kavanagh, J. F., and T. J. Truss. 1988. *Learning disabilities: Proceedings of the national conference.* Parkton, MD: York Press.

Milani-Comparetti, A., and E. Gidoni. 1967. Routine developmental examination in normal and retarded children. *Developmental Medicine and Child Neurology* 9:631-38.

Morris, S. E., and M. Dunn Klein. 1987. *Pre-feeding skills.* Tucson, AZ: Therapy Skill Builders.

Ornitz, E. M. 1974. The modulation of sensory input and motor output in autistic children. *Journal of Autism and Childhood Schizophrenia* 4:197-215.

Ornitz, E. M., and V. Honrubia. "Developmental Modulation of Vestibular-Ocular Function." In *Advances in oto-rhino-laryngology.* Vol. 41, *Neurophysiology of the vestibular system,* edited by E. Pirodda and O. Pompeiano, 36-39. New York: Karger, 1988.

Ottenbacher, K. 1978. Identifying vestibular processing dysfunction in learning disabled children. *American Journal of Occupational Therapy* 32(4):217-21.

Ottenbacher, K., A. Bundy, and M. A. Short. 1983. The development and treatment of oral-motor dysfunction: A review of clinical research. *Physical and Occupational Therapy in Pediatrics* 3(2):1-13.

Ottenbacher, K., J. Hicks, A. Roark, and J. Swinea. 1983. Oral sensorimotor therapy in the developmentally disabled: A multiple baseline study. *American Journal of Occupational Therapy* 37(8):541-47.

Paine, R. S. 1961. The early diagnosis of cerebral palsy. *Rhode Island Medical Journal* 44:522-27.

———. 1969. Early recognition of neuromotor disability in infants of low birthweight. *Developmental Medicine and Child Neurology* 11:455-59.

Paine, R. S., and T. E. Oppe. 1966. *Neurological examination of children*. Little Club Clinics in Developmental Medicine, No. 20/21. London: The National Spastics Society Medical Education and Information Unit in association with William Heinemann Medical Books.

Prechtl, H. F. 1965. Prognostic value of neurological signs in the newborn infant. *Proceedings of the Royal Society of Medicine* 58:3-4.

Prechtl, H., and D. Beintema. 1975. *The neurological examination of the full-term newborn infant*. Little Club Clinics in Developmental Medicine, No. 12. London: The National Spastics Society Medical Education and Information Unit in association with William Heinemann Medical Books.

Ruff, H. A., and K. R. Lawson. 1990. Development of sustained, focused attention in young children during free play. *Developmental Psychology* 26:85-93.

Sameroff, A. J., and R. N. Emde. 1989. *Relationship disturbances in early childhood*. New York: Basic Books.

Scherer, K. R., and P. Ekman. 1984. *Approaches to emotion*. Hillsdale, NJ: Lawrence Erlbaum Associates.

Scherzer, A. L., and I. Tscharnuter. 1982. *Early diagnosis and therapy in cerebral palsy*. New York: Marcel Dekker.

Short, M. A. 1985. Vestibular stimulation as early experience: Historical perspectives and research implications. *Physical and Occupational Therapy in Pediatrics* 5:135-52.

Sokolov, E. N. "Neuronal Models and the Orienting Reflex." In *The central nervous system and behavior,* edited by M. A. B. Brazier. New York: Josiah Macy Jr. Foundation, 1960.

Stern, D. N. 1985. *The interpersonal world of the infant*. New York: Basic Books.

Tronick, E. Z. 1989. Emotions and emotional communication in infants. *American Psychologist* 44(2):112-19.

Improve your clients' ability to accept sensory input with these materials . . .

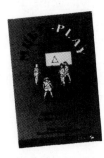

MULTI-PLAY
Sensory Activities for School Readiness
by Gerri A. Duran, OTR/L, and Sharon Klenke-Ormiston, M.A., CCC-SLP
Build on your kindergarten clients' natural play experiences to increase their school readiness. Strengthen motor skills, language, and speech with play-based multisensory activities. Plus, use this collaborative model to involve teachers in classroom carryover. **Catalog No. 4306-YTS**

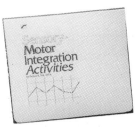

SENSORY-MOTOR INTEGRATION ACTIVITIES
by Barbara E. Fink, OTR
Help your clients improve their sensory-motor integration and development with these creative activities. You'll have more than 200 reproducible instruction sheets covering categories such as tactile, vestibular, kinesthesia, and flexion. Each activity offers a performance objective, basic procedure, measurement guidelines, and variations to help you program appropriately for the sensitivity levels of each client.
Catalog No. 4160-YTS

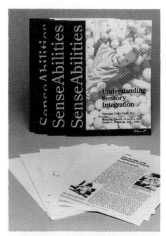

SENSEABILITIES
Understanding Sensory Integration
by Maryann Colby Trott, M.A., with Marci Laurel, M.A., CCC-SLP, and Susan L. Windeck, M.S., OTR/L
Educate parents and teachers about sensory integration with this easy-to-understand training resource. Give them practical information they can apply to real-life situations. Activities encourage children 5 to 12 years old to move across all sensory domains without realizing it! Reproduce all or part of the material including chapters on the tactile and vestibular system, therapy session, school, and more. **Catalog No. 4283-YTS**

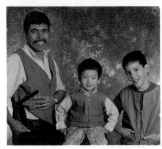

KELLIVEST®
Provide proprioceptive feedback with maximum calming deep pressure and help increase muscle tone with these weighted vests. Insert ½-, ¾-, or 1-pound weight pouches into the four interior pockets (two front, two back). Adjust the total vest weight to meet the needs of individual clients. The high positioning of the inner pockets assures the same calming deep pressure when either sitting or standing.

Small (with 4 ½-lb. weights) Catalog No. 4246-YTS
Medium (with 4 ¾-lb. weights) Catalog No. 4247-YTS
Large (with 4 1-lb weights) Catalog No. 4248-YTS
Weight Pouches available for reorder in sets of 4—
½-lb. Catalog No. 4249-YTS
¾-lb. Catalog No. 4250-YTS
1-lb. Catalog No. 4251-YTS

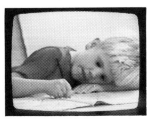

SENSORY INTEGRATION THERAPY
by Toronto Sensory Integration Study Group

This 20-minute, full-color videotape allows you to explore the unique environment of sensory integration therapy. Use it to train therapists, students, teachers, or to educate parents. The program discusses the process of SI and shows characteristics and behaviors of children with SI disorders. It also outlines target areas for therapy. Plus, a balance of therapeutic activities provides the sensory motor foundation for learning.

Catalog No. 4715-YTS

Fun-to-do activities engage children to experiment with motion . . .

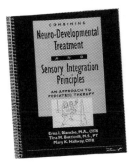

COMBINING NEURO-DEVELOPMENTAL TREATMENT AND SENSORY INTEGRATION PRINCIPLES
An Approach to Pediatric Therapy
by Erna I. Blanche, M.A., M.O.T., OTR, Tina M. Botticelli, M.S., PT, and Mary K. Hallway, OTR

Use this guide to help you combine the two most prevalent methods of treatment in pediatric therapy: Neuro-Developmental Treatment (NDT) and Sensory Integration (SI). Focus on remediating sensory and movement problems that affect the daily activities of your clients, birth to 12 years. Create an individualized therapy program that is appropriate for each client, using the techniques you find most helpful. This manual includes a discussion of both approaches, and the many benefits of combining the two. This exhaustive resource includes ample information about assessing and treating movement disorders and sensory processing disorders.

Catalog No. 4334-YTS

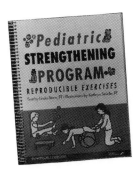

PEDIATRIC STRENGTHENING PROGRAM
Reproducible Exercises
Text by Linda Stern, PT
Illustrations by Kathryn Steidle, PT

Get your pediatric clients back on the right track with these strengthening exercises. Clients perform isolated movements and practice normal movement patterns with 108 activities. Learn feedback techniques that encourage your clients to adopt new patterns of movement. Easy-to-follow instructions and illustrations accompany each exercise and encourage participation in carryover programs. **Catalog No. 4348-YTS**

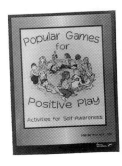

POPULAR GAMES FOR POSITIVE PLAY
Activities for Self-Awareness
by Barbara Sher, M.A., OTR

Encourage your toddler through 11-year-old clients to express and understand themselves with these easy-to-organize, no-special-materials-required games. Perform self-esteem and self-awareness activities in a context that makes learning fun. Incorporate all of these lessons into an engaging, non-competitive, no right-or-wrong context. Focus on specific motor and communication skills, or create an all-encompassing positive play plan. Lead games for individuals, pairs, small groups, or whole classes! All of the games are cross-referenced by type, and very few of them require any materials at all. **Catalog No. 4362-YTS**

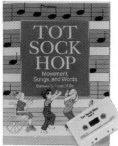

TOT SOCK HOP
Movement, Songs, and Words
by Barbara C. Trube, M.Ed.

Improve your students' gross motor, fine motor, and language skills with singing and dancing. You'll have songs, dances, rhythmic movement exercises, and speech and language activities all incorporated into one program. Meet the requirements for regular and adaptive physical education classes using OT/PT/SLP goals and objectives.

Catalog No. 4744-YTS

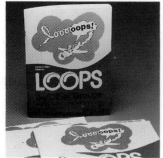

LOOPS AND OTHER GROUPS
A Kinesthetic Writing System
by Mary D. Benbow, M.S., OTR/L

Help your second-grade through high school students learn the formations of all lower-case letters in just six weeks! This writing program develops systematic steps for letter analysis and provides easy-to-remember motor and memory cues. Students learn by using four groups of letters which share common movement patterns—Clock Climbers, Kite Strings, Loop Group, and Hills and Valleys.

Catalog No. 4189-YTS

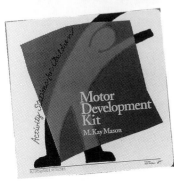

MOTOR DEVELOPMENT KIT
Activity Sessions for Children
by M. Kay Mason

Help your students with motor delays or difficulties improve their skills using this motor development program. Working through seven activity stations, your school-age students will increase muscle tone, correct posture, and build confidence. Each station addresses basic concepts that encourage the development of a wide range of motor, cognitive, and language skills. Within each station, activities vary in difficulty. Materials needed for the activities are included in the kit or can easily be made from everyday items.

Catalog No. 4337-YTS

For more information on these practical resources, please call 1-800-228-0752.

- -

ORDER FORM

Ship to:

INSTITUTION: _____

NAME: _____

OCCUPATION/DEPT: _____

ADDRESS: _____

CITY:_____ STATE:_____ ZIP: _____

Please check here if this is a permanent address change.

Telephone No._____ ☐ work ☐ home

Payment Options:

☐ Bill me.   ☐ My check is enclosed.

☐ My purchase order is enclosed. P.O.#_____

☐ Charge to my credit card.   (Net 30 days)

   ☐ VISA ☐ MasterCard ☐ American Express

Card No. ☐☐☐☐☐☐☐☐☐☐☐☐☐☐☐☐

Expiration Date: Month_____ Year _____

Signature_____

Prices are in U.S. dollars. Payment must be made in U.S. funds only.

QTY.	CAT. #	TITLE	AMOUNT

- If your account is not currently listed as "tax exempt," applicable destination charges will be added to your invoice.
- Orders are shipped by United Parcel Service (UPS) unless otherwise requested. If another delivery service is required, please specify.
- For regular delivery service, your order will be charged 5% handling plus actual shipping charges.
- We occasionally backorder items temporarily out of stock. If you do not accept backorders, please tell us on your purchase order or on this form.

MONEY-BACK GUARANTEE
You'll have up to 90 days of risk-free evaluation of the products you ordered. If you're not completely satisfied with any product, we'll pick it up within the 90 days and refund the full purchase price! *No questions asked!*

FOR PHONE ORDERS
Call 1-800-228-0752. Please have your credit card and/or institutional purchase order information ready.
Monday–Friday 7AM–7PM Central Time
Voice or TDD 1-800-723-1318
FAX 1-800-232-1223

Send your order to:

Therapy Skill Builders
a division of The Psychological Corporation
555 Academic Court / San Antonio, Texas 78204-2498